CBD

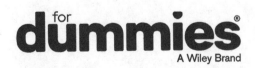

A Wiley Brand

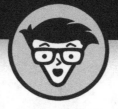

CBD

by Blair Lauren Brown

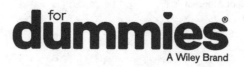

A Wiley Brand

CBD For Dummies®

Published by: **John Wiley & Sons, Inc.,** 111 River Street, Hoboken, NJ 07030-5774, www.wiley.com

Copyright © 2021 by John Wiley & Sons, Inc., Hoboken, New Jersey

Published simultaneously in Canada

For general information on our other products and services, please contact our Customer Care Department within the U.S. at 877-762-2974, outside the U.S. at 317-572-3993, or fax 317-572-4002. For technical support, please visit https://hub.wiley.com/community/support/dummies.

Wiley publishes in a variety of print and electronic formats and by print-on-demand. Some material included with standard print versions of this book may not be included in e-books or in print-on-demand. If this book refers to media such as a CD or DVD that is not included in the version you purchased, you may download this material at http://booksupport.wiley.com. For more information about Wiley products, visit www.wiley.com.

Library of Congress Control Number: 2021939760

ISBN 978-1-119-67472-6 (pbk); ISBN 978-1-119-67458-0 (ebk); ISBN 978-1-119-67480-1 (ebk)

Manufactured in the United States of America

SKY10027771_062421

Contents at a Glance

Recipes at a Glance

Table of Contents

Introduction

Getting high isn't the only reason to dip your toe into hemp or cannabis-derived products. Cannabidiol (CBD), a non-psychoactive compound found in the cannabis plant, has proven to be a powerful medicine for dozens of different ailments. From rheumatoid arthritis to menopause, CBD is proving to be a missing link in formerly dire and nearly untreatable medical circumstances. And less bleak circumstances, like a lack of sexual excitement or lowered libido, are also being investigated as conditions that CBD can remedy. No matter the source of your curiosity, *CBD For Dummies* can help you leap from uninformed consumer to confident and competent CBD advocate.

About This Book

Many people think of themselves as cannabis experts, but their knowledge base may come from faulty sources. Movies like *Pineapple Express* and *How High* create narratives that the plant is dangerous or magical. And your old college roommate who has a friend of a friend who bakes pot cookies probably isn't a top-tier source, either.

This book focuses on the ins and outs of CBD, with its psychedelic cousin THC playing more of a minor role. My goal is to give you a foundation to make informed decisions as a consumer on how to treat ailments (specifically found in Part 3 of this book) and improve your life with the help of CBD. If you're more advanced than a complete newbie, that's great! You'll find some sections to be intuitive or obvious. I also dive into a series of recipes (found in Part 4) so that you can start using CBD in your home, in formats that are familiar, with recipes for facial products, and others for edible treats for you and even your pets. I hope to also give you new insights into the cannabis industry, relevant legislation, medicinal history and applications, and even recreational mediums.

Note: As you build your repertoire of cannabis knowledge, remember that none of the advice in this book can replace a consultation with a medical professional. Additionally, although I explore many different delivery methods, the CBD vehicle that will give you the best experience is completely up to you. You're not a carbon copy, and CBD isn't one-size-fits-all.

Foolish Assumptions

I've made a few assumptions about you as I've written this book:

>> You want to try CBD and are curious about alternative medicines. You know that you prefer a more naturopathic approach to wellness and are hoping to transition from traditional pills and potions to a more holistic solution.

>> You recognize that CBD is a huge industry with many different opinions and options on how to get started. You're willing to take the time to tailor your CBD treatment method to your lifestyle and other unique points of consideration.

>> You're willing to form your own opinions, using diligent research and soliciting credible consultations. You know that the only expert on your body is you and accept that no rules apply everywhere without exception.

>> You realize that all that glitters isn't gold. You recognize that, as in any industry, some CBD companies are more reputable or trustworthy than others.

Icons Used in This Book

Throughout the book, I use a handful of icons to point out various types of information. Here's what they are and what they mean:

Think of this icon as the little star you may draw next to important items on your grocery list. It marks areas that are great reference points to commit to memory.

This icon points out tidbits of information that are interesting but not essential. If you're in a hurry or into speed-reading, you can skip paragraphs marked with this icon and still be just fine.

The Tip icon is for actionable blurbs of advice and sometimes brand or product recommendations.

This one is essentially a "Slippery When Wet" road sign. Use this icon to avoid unnecessary pitfalls.

Beyond the Book

The Cheat Sheet is an awesome way to explore bite-sized information on some of the most important points about getting acquainted with CBD. This little freebie is definitely worth a gander.

To access this Cheat Sheet, simply go to www.dummies.com and search for "CBD For Dummies Cheat Sheet."

Where to Go from Here

The great thing about this book is that you can start anywhere. Just mosey on over to the table of contents or index to identify your topic of interest and begin reading.

If you're not quite sure what CBD is and why it may positively impact your body in a supplementary form, Chapters 2 and 3 give you a complete overview of CBD and what its functions are.

On the other hand, if you feel like you want to get a sense of how to find the right delivery method for you, go straight to Chapter 7.

On the other hand (you've got three hands, right?), if you want to get started whipping up some customized recipes, your best bet is to visit Part 4.

Whatever the case, please approach the book with a sense of open-mindedness and enjoyment. Remember, you're here to have fun and to get great information. It's go time!

1
Looking into CBD

Beef up your CBD knowledge, vocabulary, and technique.

Define CBD and become familiar with the different parts of the hemp plant.

Dig into the four pillars of CBD relief and the pros and cons of CBD supplementation.

Investigate the different layers of CBD extraction and the different products it can yield.

IN THIS CHAPTER

» Separating CBD fact from fiction

» Trying out a couple of treatment methods

» Recognizing some of CBD's medical benefits

» Understanding the history and future of CBD laws and acceptance

Chapter 1

Updating Attitudes toward Cannabis and CBD

C BD is one of hundreds of naturally occurring chemical compounds in the cannabis plant. Because that plant has long had a sordid history in the Western world, CBD carries a perception of danger and illicit behavior. The reality is that CBD offers many potential therapeutic benefits in and of itself without the inebriating, or "high," effects that give cannabis its reputation.

The everyday consumer and even some of the canna-curious find themselves butting up against myths that are a function of the times. In this chapter, I unpack the differences between the different types of cannabis and how CBD got its (not entirely fair) reputation. I also delve into its practical uses and medical benefits, as well as legality issues surrounding CBD. After reading this chapter, you'll become a pro at separating CBD rumors from realities. (For a deeper dive into what CBD actually is, flip to Chapter 2.)

Debunking Myths about CBD

The list of rumors and myths about CBD is long because the cannabis plant is new in Western applications and the research is young. You may have heard that CBD is illegal because it comes from the cannabis plant. Or perhaps you've heard that it comes from hemp, but you're only familiar with hemp as a source of fabric. You may have heard that CBD is a snake oil, made popular only by the placebo effect. On the other hand, maybe you've been told that CBD really can cure it *all*.

Table 1-1 provides a quick overview of some common myths surrounding CBD as well as the actual facts. In the following sections, I talk about some of these myths in more detail.

TABLE 1-1   **Separating Common CBD Fact from Fiction**

Fiction	Fact
CBD is a Schedule 1 narcotic drug, so there is no research.	Formal, government-sanctioned research, as well as a host of anecdotal evidence, does exist. It is also "descheduled."
CBD is snake oil and a scam.	CBD has plenty of legitimate applications.
CBD as an industry is chock-full of discrepancies and is thus unsafe.	CBD hasn't been shown to physically harm anyone.
CBD can cure anything.	CBD has been shown to help some conditions; like anything, results vary.

CURE: A LOADED WORD

The myth of all myths is that CBD can cure anything. *Cure* is a word you don't often hear in any kind of medicine because it implies that whatever caused the symptoms is no longer there. That's a hard threshold to reach. Results inevitably vary from body to body, so claiming a cure is difficult. Anecdotal evidence and the FDA's new approved CBD anti-seizure medicine, Epidiolex, indicate that CBD has provided a lot of relief to a diverse group of people. And as a recognized figure in the space, I have heard of plenty of successful applications of CBD across individuals and with companies developing products.

Understanding where some of the uncertainty about CBD comes from

The CBD molecule is found largely in the cannabis plant. However, new evidence suggests that it also appears in an invasive species of pine tree. Early research suggests that many plants contain a host of other molecules that mimic the functions and properties of CBD.

From a federal standpoint, cannabis containing THC is illegal. *Hemp cannabis*, which contains 0.3 percent or less THC content by dry weight, has been allowed for use with various FDA disclaimers on use practices. CBD is derived from hemp cannabis. (Head to the later section "Looking at the Legality Surrounding CBD" for more on legal specifics.)

REMEMBER

CBD used to be lumped in with THC-dominant cannabis as a Schedule 1 narcotic drug. Because of that classification, research was limited to federal institutions (or abroad) — no private studies. So much of the existing research available is limited to the interests of the federal government; relevant information isn't very accessible, leading to the widespread fear that CBD is unsafe.

TECHNICAL STUFF

CBD was actually isolated and discovered as far back as 1940.

The declassification of hemp cannabis cleared the way for the allowance of CBD in products. Retailers clamored to get their hands on the new "it-girl" ingredient. This frenzy incited a rush to the marketplace with everything from tinctures and balms to CBD-infused pillows. Little regulation on the natural and supplement market in the United States meant few barriers to entry.

As knowledge of CBD's uses as a supplement grew, companies began churning out long lists of claims about its supposed benefits: pain relief, better sleep, reduction of wrinkles, cell turnover — the list goes on. Some of these claims were merely that — claims. Some were and are based on private studies and years of experience. Ultimately, some CBD products may be scams; as with any new industry, companies with little integrity try to make a quick buck.

But it's not all smoke and mirrors. CBD has lots of legitimate uses as natural medicine. Interestingly enough, the United States even holds patents (almost 40, in fact) on cannabis. One of the most acknowledged and talked about is on cannabis as a neuroprotective as well as an anti-inflammatory and antioxidative agent.

HOLDING CBD PRODUCTS TO A HIGHER (DOUBLE) STANDARD

Consumers today are more knowledgeable and empowered in their ingredient knowledge than ever, but they don't necessarily hold all plant-derived ingredients to the same standard. Take tea tree oil. It first came to the Western product market as an antibacterial; soon, it was in everything from soaps to toothpaste to honey. People took it at face value and consumed it in abundance. Now compare that approach to the hoops consumers want CBD products to jump through. They want to look at certificates of analysis (COAs) and know the location of the farm. I don't know about you, but I don't know exactly where the tea tree in my toothpaste comes from, and I'm an over-the-top kind of principled buyer of products. Most consumers didn't even know what a COA was before the cannabis market opened up. The difference? Tea tree oil doesn't come with the stigma of having been classified as an illicit substance.

CBD is not a cure-all, but neutralizes many difficult symptoms

The early phases of CBD in the consumer marketplace have led to a host of one-size-fits-all forms of CBD. The most common offering is full-spectrum tinctures. Other varieties include capsules, powders, balms, and salves. Some companies are creating very targeted ingredients with CBD, and still others are creating products with CBD and other ingredients designed to address specific conditions.

Research and anecdotal evidence for the many uses of CBD continues to expand. Broad applications showed success in inflammatory relief, and evidence indicates CBD can address topical conditions like eczema, scarring, and acne. Now researchers are testing extra functions such as antimicrobial and antifungal qualities.

More than 50 percent of Americans suffer from chronic pain, sleep, and anxiety conditions, and CBD can help there as well. The reported internal benefits of CBD range from help with chronic and acute pain to stress reduction and relief from depression and sleeplessness. Other applications include gut health, mental fog, arthritis, exercise fatigue, and more. The formal medical uses are limited because of CBD's novelty, but they're showing incredible promise.

The most significant medical applications to date are related to epilepsy and seizures. A pharmaceutical company created the drug Epidiolex, which is designed to treat a severe seizure condition and has been proven to limit the severity, duration, and frequency of condition-related seizures. Researchers are exploring other pharmaceutical uses in more depth, including a host of neurological conditions that have stumped the drug industry and healthcare professionals for generations.

TIP

If you don't know what you're treating, quantifying results is hard. In Chapter 7, I cover how to know the difference in form, ingredient, and condition to ensure CBD products you choose can serve your particular needs. Part 3 also covers all sorts of ailments and conditions and how CBD may be able to help.

Applying and Ingesting CBD

CBD is not just a one-trick pony, or a one-form pony, for lack of better analogies. That's a common misconception that needs to be corrected. Many people think that the whole-plant form reigns superior for consumption. CBD cannabis flower, the true whole-plant form, is beautiful. The host of plant chemicals contained inside can address a broad spectrum of conditions and side effects. However, it is not the best form of CBD if it is not a form that works for you.

REMEMBER

When CBD is processed into an extract, there are varying degrees of so-called purity. The purest form that you could get is CBD-isolate, which contains nothing but pure CBD. When you subscribe to the whole-plant method, isolate is off the table for you. Instead, you will only look at products such as full-spectrum extracts that contain the whole plant. Subscribing to a clinical and impersonal definition of rightness is limiting. The narrow perception of CBD as solely a full-spectrum extract prohibits the perception of its diversity of application and opportunities. Let's not pigeonhole CBD!

Uncovering the right form for you is a bit of an art. And while I go into some of the details of the form factors later in this section, it's helpful to go into a more specific approach to conditions and side-effects and evaluate the "right" form factor from there. As a start, read through this chapter, and if you find you want to jump straight to the deeper information on form factors, hop to Chapter 7. Topicals are discussed in more depth in Chapter 14, more specifically as they relate to skincare. Chapter 21 offers a broader overview of the "why" coupled with what form.

As an all-natural remedy, CBD has been declared effective as both a topical and ingestible treatment. The condition you're treating ultimately determines the best form to use. A topical application of CBD is best for localized or acute pain, which can be caused by a bonk or a bruise. Examples of topical products include body oils and lotions. Ingestible forms of CBD are best for chronic pain conditions. The following sections break down the basics of topical and ingestible treatments.

REMEMBER

New findings have led not only to more sophisticated combinations of CBD but also to adaptations of CBD from its more raw extracts into complex formulations. These cutting-edge creations are versatile and can be topical or ingestible.

Applying CBD to the skin

Topical applications of CBD can treat both external and internal issues. The external treatments don't absorb beyond the top three layers of the skin. These options — ranging from lotions, salves, creams, and balms to oils — are prevalent in both the skincare and the pain markets. The list of benefits here is particularly long. The primary targets are inflammatory skin conditions, including dry skin, itchy irritations, dehydration, and rough patches and cracks. CBD is also an antioxidant and thus is touted for protecting skin from the signs of aging as well as addressing more difficult skin conditions such as eczema, psoriasis, and acne.

Treating internal conditions topically is a little more complicated. The skin is the largest external organ; it serves as a protective barrier that either allows or prevents substances from reaching the bloodstream. Topicals designed to treat external (surface-level) skin conditions don't need to penetrate below the outermost layer of the skin, but to take care of internal complaints, CBD must reach the bloodstream. That's where transdermal agents come in.

Topical applications for internal benefits are known as *transdermal agents* (or *transdermals*). Transdermals require a *penetrating agent* — something that damages the skin in a microirritation. This microirritation allows the active agents to pass through the skin and into the bloodstream. Think of those pain relief patches that seem to change temperature. The "heat" is the penetrating agent (the cooling is there to mediate the heat sensation). The CBD market has only briefly approached transdermals, but a host of companies offer patches specifically for localized pain.

Eating or ingesting CBD

When choosing an edible/ingestible form of CBD, you have two important considerations:

» Bioavailability (the amount of a substance that reaches the bloodstream)

» Onset time (how quickly the CBD takes effect)

Sublingual applications (applied under the tongue) are the fastest-acting and most calibrated of CBD offerings next to smoking. Chewable tablets like mints; gums; and dissolvable strips, tinctures, teas, and oral sprays all fall under the sublingual category because they're in your mouth for a while. And the sublingual oil market is one of the most dominant categories in ingestible CBD.

Sublingual action is made possible through the medicine meeting the mucous membrane under the tongue. The membrane and connective tissue under the tongue contain capillaries (the smallest and largest concentration of blood vessels). On sublingual administration, the medicine dissolves and is absorbed into the bloodstream through the tiny network of blood vessels. The faster the medicine hits the bloodstream, the faster the onset. The least obstacles in the way of the medicine reaching the bloodstream means the largest amount of bioavailability.

Other forms of edibles (like chocolates, candies, or gummies) have the disadvantage of having to travel through the gut for absorption. The problem is that they encounter quite a few warriors (such as stomach acid) along the way, which challenges their bioavailability and onset time. Supplements like capsules and powders, and anything else you may swallow, struggle with the same obstacles. On the flip side, they have the comfort of a more traditional supplement market.

CBD: The New Treatment of Choice?

"Illegal, illicit narcotic banned by the government for over 40 years is now making its way into the hands of the severely ill and having incredible benefits!" I just made that headline up, but it sounds like something you could've read in all the frenzy over CBD since it was declassified in 2018. (See the later section "Looking at the Legality Surrounding CBD" for that move.) CBD has the appeal of an affordable, accessible miracle, but the frenzy is just a fad. For CBD to really have long-term staying power, we need to see maximum benefits and efficacy in the CBD medicine space. That may require a few more years to apply research. We need patient-backed outcome studies to attest to successes in a uniform and repeatable way.

So yes, for now, this is just a fad that requires a lot of work on behalf of the customer for positive outcomes. That or a really good friend, or book, which might be able to provide some guidance to start the process of sorting through the weeds. (No pun intended.)

Providing a natural alternative to Western healthcare

The timing of the legalization of CBD couldn't have been better. In this day and age, people are more and more disillusioned with traditional Western healthcare and are therefore looking for alternative remedies to legitimately heal what ails them. The Western focus tends to treat the symptoms; natural and alternative medicines tend to focus on the whole and the underlying causes or roots of an ailment.

CBD falls into that natural category right now. Its compatibility with the human body is truly remarkable. The introduction of CBD and other cannabinoids addresses a general balance that can potentially systematically ease symptoms caused by a core root condition. It may even address the condition in some cases.

And it's proving to be quite successful for some in the experiential phases of exploring CBD as a personal remedy. As the science and uses evolve, more targeted remedies and more customer education will become available.

The combination of the minimal applicable science and widespread fear about CBD has made way for the general population to take charge of their education about the plant, the chemicals, and what they could be using. This self-empowerment model is unlike anything else the natural health space has seen regarding a single ingredient.

Move over, opiates: Considering CBD for treating pain

One of the more promising areas of study and usage for CBD is pain. The chemical is a nonaddictive alternative to opiates because of its anti-inflammatory action. CBD expedites the body's inflammatory response system and alleviates pain sensations while simultaneously speeding up recovery.

Opiates tend to be a pharmacological tool applied to both acute and chronic pain, but they present more of a problem with the latter. Pain that persists for long periods can be harder to treat because it has perpetual effects on the neurological state. The result: more opiate use over longer durations. This prolonged use comes with a host of side effects, including dependency.

The focus of opiates is pain relief specifically; think of them as a single blade. CBD is more like a multi-tool for pain.

If the end result is relief either way, and one opportunity presents fewer side effects and less risk of dependency, the winner seems clear. All the hows and whys of this are explored in more depth on a condition-by-condition basis in Part 3.

Looking at the Legality Surrounding CBD

CBD is now a legal extract from a hemp plant, so long as no THC is present in the product. (In some cases, 0.3 percent or less THC is acceptable.) The task now is unpacking the unnecessary criminalization of the plant. Coming back from the implications of being a Schedule 1 drug is challenging, but the future of cannabis is bright.

Breaking down the criminalization of CBD

In the 1930s, cannabis became a regulated substance and then a prohibited substance — not the kind of upgrade you want. The law made absolutely no separation between cannabis with THC and hemp cannabis.

Why this change happened is an interesting question. Theories range from a paper commission to a conglomerate of businesses out to serve only themselves. (At the time, hemp was used and grown for industrial purposes only, from paper to fabric production to protein as a food source.) Others say the federal government specifically intended to villainize a population of people who were using cannabis. And still another theory supports the two theories combined, suggesting that the politics and corporate interests were intertwined. Plenty of evidence seems to support the theory of villanization. In fact, contemporary dissection of the War on Drugs reveals the U.S. administration's fabrication and popularization of stories of black and brown populations using marijuana and becoming super villains. Regardless, the implications of the history of cannabis continue to affect people — maybe you, maybe your neighbors and friends — today.

Changing attitudes and changing laws

The U.S. federal government declassified hemp and hemp-derived CBD in 2018, leading to a steady flow of hemp CBD products into the marketplace. Scientists and researchers are now allowed access previously given only to government organizations. Government cannabis and hemp flowers for research came from an extremely limited pool of resources. Only minimal viable information was accessible, which limited expansion efforts for both public acceptance and product development.

REMEMBER

The longer nongovernment scientists have access, the more information the public will see and the more familiar and more comfortable people will be as consumers. So the more consumers vote with their dollars by adopting CBD products, the better the evolution of quality and then the application will become.

Moving toward new understanding

CBD as a chemical has only just been extracted (excuse the pun) from the common assumption that it's going to get you high like its cannabinoid cousin THC. For such myths to be put to bed for good, a few things need to happen:

>> The facts about hemp cannabis and CBD need to trickle down from the science community to the lay population.

>> The whole plant needs to be removed from any state of regulation.

>> People everywhere need to think long and hard about their existing beliefs in light of these new changes.

IN THIS CHAPTER

» **Digging into hemp**

» **Understanding what's in hemp and how those components work together**

» **Feeling out hemp strains**

» **Discovering other plants that contain CBD and CBD-like substances**

» **Comparing natural and synthetic CBD**

Chapter **2**

Examining CBD Itself

Without understanding the whole plant, it's hard to get a proper picture of CBD. I love the idea of getting the entire story of the plant by, *you guessed it,* using the whole plant as medicine. It requires a special level of attunement and sensitivity to engage with cannabis in this way. When I say that the relationship to the plant spirit is part of the medicine, the general plant medicine community is in agreement. To better honor this relationship, the plant must be as close to its natural state as possible. And to clarify, my statement is not just limited to form but also applies to cultivation and use.

In this chapter, I explore the plant and plants (yes, I said *plants,* plural) containing CBD. I also walk you through the components and complements of the whole plant and their relationship to CBD. And finally, I introduce you to synthetic CBD.

Meeting the Mother of All CBD Sources

Because of hemp's relation to the cannabis plant as a whole, differentiating them is important. Cannabis and hemp both come from the same plant species, *Cannabis sativa,* but their chemical makeups and respective uses vary. Hemp is associated with industrial use, with cultivation focusing on the stalks. Cannabis is the one often referred to as marijuana. It has been cultivated and revered (as well as criminalized and stigmatized) for the psychoactive properties found in its flowers, also called the *buds*.

The hemp plant has a vast history and myriad standalone virtues that I explore in the following sections.

Delving into the long history of hemp

Plants in the cannabis family are widely referred to as "weed" because of the way they grow abundantly with little attention. They can break up soil, survive in varied climates, and adapt quickly. Historically, then, hemp has been easy to cultivate and therefore lent itself to proliferation. (Of course, intentional cultivation in very controlled environments to support and bring out specific characteristics also happens.)

The history of the hemp plant spans cultures and generations. You can find well over 22,000 recorded uses for hemp seeds, stalks, and flowers (but I don't recommend looking for all of them). The applications throughout time may surpass that of any other plant. Here are just a few across time and continents:

>> Allegedly, Buddhist texts dating back to the second and third centuries CE were printed on hemp-dominant paper.

>> Hemp cloth from 8000 BCE was discovered in what was once ancient Mesopotamia.

>> Chinese educational texts from 500 CE teach hemp cultivation techniques for making cloth.

>> King Henry VIII required landowners in 1535 to grow at least a quarter acre of hemp so that the supply would be sufficient for canvas production for ship sails. This record is just one account of Europe's heavy reliance on hemp-derived canvas fiber and rope.

>> In 1938, *Popular Mechanics* hailed hemp as the new billion-dollar crop, and Americans were incentivized by the government to grow the plant abundantly. (Shortly thereafter, they were then penalized by the same governing body for growing it abundantly. I touch on this topic briefly in Chapter 1.)

Identifying the parts of the hemp plant

Here are the essential features of the hemp plant; you can see them in Figure 2-1:

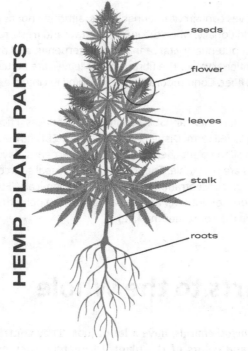

HEMP PLANT PARTS

- seeds
- flower
- leaves
- stalk
- roots

FIGURE 2-1:
The hemp plant.

Courtesy of Poplar

>> **Seeds:** Hemp seeds are generally considered a superfood, chock full of protein and fiber. They also contain a host of other medically appreciated benefits. You can find minerals, healthy fats such as omega-3s, and vitamins including magnesium and vitamins B6 and E in hemp seeds; all of these are essential to a healthy system. Fuel, food, and oil are also derivatives of the seeds when they can be processed in large quantities.

>> **Stalks:** The stalks are the most vital part of the plant for fiber production; they're where the ropes, canvas, and paper I mention in the preceding section ultimately hail from. The fiber is an ingredient in compost and can be used for animal bedding and for insulation purposes. The more hemp is cultivated in modern times, the more uses are starting to pop up across industries.

Because of the interest in creating fiber, hemp plants are grown tightly packed in fields so they stretch to the sun, creating long stalks much like bamboo.

TECHNICAL
STUFF

>> **Roots:** The roots are incredible *bioremediators,* meaning they can help extract toxins from the ground around them. They can also break up troublesome hard soil, making it more manageable. They contain an incredible concentration of the healing compounds in hemp.

>> **Leaves:** Hemp leaves contain vital cannabinoids, although not as plentifully as the flowers do. Additionally, when the leaves are raw and fresh, rather than dried, they contain potentially vital cannabinoids, terpenes, and other properties of nutritional value. The fibrous hemp leaves are better served up as edible nutrient fiber. Contemporary uses including juicing to extract these vital nutrients.

>> **Flower:** Hemp, like its other cannabis counterpart, produces a flower (the bud) when grown to full term. Dispensaries sell it as a CBD flower. Hemp flowers are rich in all the plant chemicals, including terpenes, flavonoids, and cannabinoids, and are smokable. They're also the principal source for extracts because of their high concentration of potent plant chemicals. (Fun fact: The hemp flower is more sought-after and has a higher price point than a lot of the THC flowers on the consumer market.)

Explaining the Parts to the Whole

Plant chemicals, or *phytochemicals,* have a lot of jobs. They contribute to the flavors, tastes, smells, and colors of the plant. Ultimately, they exist to help the survival of the plant itself.

The functions of plant chemicals — microbial resistance, reduction of inflammatory response, fungal protection, and more — are transferrable. That's why you're supposed to eat so many vegetables: Phytochemicals can dually protect plants and humans from unhealthy risks. (So, spoiler alert, your mother was right — eat your leafy greens!) Major plant chemicals in hemp include terpenes, flavonoids (color and flavor contributors), more than 120 cannabinoids, and the enzymes that make the chemical reactions possible.

Debating the benefits of using the whole plant versus the sum of its parts

The *entourage effect* is the predominant philosophy in the world of hemp and marijuana. Many believe that you need to have the whole plant (or all the pieces of the plant in their respective ratios, as they originate in a single plant) to get the most beneficial therapeutic effects.

That said, generations and cultures around the world have harnessed different pieces of all plants for different purposes. For example, kava plants are prized for their roots, which have intensely calming effects. Folk remedies tout the benefits of certain plants for their ability to heal certain parts of the human body. They often equate a plant's physical resemblance to a specific body part to the plant's use as a specialized remedy for that body part. And because science has evolved to be able to study the realities of those applications, more knowledge about the uses of the pieces is available than ever before.

REMEMBER

Because prohibition has limited studies on the hemp plant as a whole and its parts, whether using the whole plant is "better" is unclear.

Appreciating all the cannabinoids in the hemp plant

Cannabinoids are the chemicals most specific to the hemp and cannabis plants because they're almost unduplicated in any other plant. More than 120 cannabinoids occur naturally in the hemp (*Cannabis sativa L.*) plant; this book focuses on CBD, but others are certainly worth a visit.

Here are the essential chemicals you need to know:

>> **Cannabidiol (CBD):** CBD is the most abundant cannabinoid in the hemp plant; it's recognized for its anti-inflammatory, pain relief, antimicrobial, and antifungal properties, among others.

REMEMBER

   CBD is also non-inebriating. Just a reminder.

>> **Tetrahydrocannabinol (THC):** THC is the cannabinoid known for its illicit history, all thanks to its psychoactive nature. Medically, it's gaining acclaim for its pain relief properties, making it an exciting candidate for treating pain conditions.

>> **Cannabichromene (CBC):** CBC has been wildly less studied, but it may lend itself chronic pain relief because of its ability to block the perception of pain.

>> **Cannabinol (CBN):** CBN is what you get when THC degenerates from long-term exposure to oxygen. Studies show that it may help treat insomnia and other sleep disorders because of its effects on certain brain receptors.

>> **Cannabigerol (CBG):** The medical implications of CBG are actually quite exciting. Cultivation for CBG is on the rise thanks to hopes of treating conditions from digestive disorders to eye disease.

Exploring terpenes and flavonoids

Terpenes are present in many life forms — around 20,000 plants and animals. They're a major player in the cannabis plant because hundreds appear in such high concentrations.

GETTING MORE FAMILIAR WITH TERPENES

With all this talk about terpenes, how about a look at some of the more common terpenes? The following chart represents some of the better-known terpenes that can be found in cannabis, hemp, and a host of other botanicals. Beyond naming the terpenes, I also outline the effects each terpene has on the body and the associated medical benefits. The aroma is one of the most identifying characteristics of a terpene, and sometimes, just by smelling a plant, you can tell the terpene profile, so just for fun, I have included the scent and a few other plants where you can find the terpene. Take a look at the chart, then test your nose on the mentioned plants.

TERPENE CHARACTERISTIC CHART

	EFFECTS	MEDICAL BENEFITS	AROMAS	FOUND IN
LINALOOL	sedating, calming	can help with insomnia, stress, depression, anxiety, pain, convulsions	floral, citrus spice	cannabis, lavender, citrus, laurel, birch, rosewood
PINENE	memory retention, alertness	can reduce inflammation and help with asthma	sharp, sweet, pine	cannabis, pine needles, conifers, sage
HUMULENE	suppresses appetite	anti-inflammatory, anti-bacterial, pain relief	woody, earthy	cannabis, hops, coriander
LIMONENE	enhances properties of other terpenes, elevated mood, stress relief	anti-depression, anti-anxiety, antifungal, can help with gastric reflux	citrus, lemon, orange	cannabis, citrus rinds, juniper, peppermint
MYRCENE	sedating, relaxing, enhances THC's psychoactivity	antiseptic, anti-bacterial, antifungal, anti-inflammatory	musk, cloves, herbal, citrus	cannabis, mango, thyme, citrus, lemongrass, bay leaves
BETA-CARYOPHYLLENE	anxiety and pain relief	antioxidant, anti-inflammatory, pain relief, can help with muscle spasms, insomnia relief	pepper, wood, spice	cannabis, pepper, cloves, hops, basil, oregano
GERANIOL	relaxation with mental alertness, pain reduction	antibacterial, antifungal	rose	cannabis, rose, palmarose, citronella, geranium, lemon
EUGENOL	calm, relaxing mental effect, may improve focus, aphrodisiac	itching relief, antibacterial, antifungal, anesthetic properties, pain relief	clove, spice	cannabis, clove, nutmeg, cinnamon, basil, bay leaf

Courtesy of Poplar

Terpenes are also referred to as terpenoids, but they aren't the same thing. *Terpenoids* are an aged and oxidized version of a terpene.

Terpenes have a lot of functions in plants. They can protect a plant from disease and act as an antimicrobial, antifungal, or antibacterial agent, and they do the same in their extract form. Thyme, for instance, has high concentrations of thymol, known for its antibacterial properties. It's quite efficient as a cleaning agent — it's actually the active ingredient in a popular brand of natural cleaning products.

Terpenes are recognizable because of their highly aromatic profiles. Essential oils actually contain high concentrations of terpenes! Aromatherapy recognizes the properties of these terpenes and takes advantage of certain aromas to address specific conditions and ailments. In the same vein, cannabis is becoming widely recognized for its ability to address many conditions and ailments. So smoking a spliff isn't so far removed from the practice of aromatherapy.

If the name doesn't say it all, flavonoids contribute to the flavor and the smell of plants. They also help with cell signaling and the antioxidant effects in the body.

Looking at enzymes and the value of the other plant molecules

Enzymes, simply put, are instigators. They're protein molecules that catalyze or start chemical reactions. They're responsible for functionality in an organism — in this case, cannabis. Enzymes do the heavy lifting not just in the plant kingdom but with humans as well. They're a vital piece for interaction with your endocannabinoid system.

Investigating the Hemp Strains and Varieties

If you aren't a botanist, plant varieties and strains may be new concepts for you. (If you are a botanist, this topic shouldn't strain you.) The difference is in the *propagation* (breeding) process:

>> **Variety:** Plant *varieties* are created through *sexual propagation,* which means the plant specimen was bred naturally from its parent's stock. Hemp specifically is created through the sexual propagation of hemp seeds.

>> **Strain:** *Strains* are an *asexual propagation* of the plant through cloning. The cloning process takes cuttings of what's commonly known as a *mother plant* and develops the same genetic profile in a repeatable fashion.

I focus on strains over varieties for CBD consumption and medicinal use. The possibility of controlling genetic outcomes is crucial for creating consistent medicinal benefits, and that genetic control comes from the cloning process.

Almost universally, hemp strains contain calming or relaxing properties. CBD lends itself to a feeling of physical relaxation. The combination of other plant chemicals, namely terpenes, in a particular strain is what causes the psychological effects you experience when you consume it. (Flip to the earlier section "Exploring terpenes and flavonoids" for more on terpenes.) Terpene profiles across strains can vary dramatically from calming to energizing.

I explore these categories more in the following sections. The key here is choosing a strain that's high in CBD and low in THC, which is the defining characteristic of a CBD strain.

I mention a few classic strain names in the following sections, but homing in on the percentage of cannabinoids and terpenes is really more important. These two traits are much like a fingerprint. They're going to be the best identifier of strain characteristics. Because of the diversity of breeding and cultivation that occurs from grower to grower and retailer to retailer, focusing on strain names isn't always the best approach.

Checking out calming strains

Calming strains have higher concentrations of the following calming terpenes:

>> Linalool

>> Myrcene

>> Limonene

Look for these options in the terpene profiles of your CBD hemp flower or distillates.

If you're looking at CBD as a remedy for stress and anxiety, make sure the strains you consume contain almost no THC. The "high" feeling of THC can be associated with paranoia and anxiety.

TIP

Remedy, ACDC, Lifter, and Charlotte's Web are a few of the more popular, widely available options.

Recognizing refreshing and revitalizing strains

Refreshing strains have uplifting and clarifying terpene profiles. In a sense, these profiles are similar to the calming terpenes in the preceding section but also include other terpenes like pinene and beta-caryophyllene. You can actually smell a more vibrant terpene profile in these types of strains.

TIP

Bubba Kush and Elektra are great for harnessing your energy and feeling energized but not sedated.

Lifting and elevating some energizing strains

Many people used to look for a sativa strain (over an indica strain) for uplifting effects. But those cheerful, energetic feelings actually come from the terpene levels, and thus, the terms indica and sativa, while they are quite new sounding to those new to cannabis, are actually seeing their way out of the conversation. The most energizing strains have valencene, pinene, and beta-caryophyllene.

TIP

Harlequin, Harle-Tsu, Sour Space Candy, Lifter, and Frosted Kush are a few of the more recognized strains for a pick-me-up.

Finding CBD and Similar Chemicals in Other Plants

The cannabis plant isn't the only source of CBD or its effects. An invasive pine tree also has CBD in its bark, and various plants contain a host of *cannabimimetics*, chemicals that interact with the body's endocannabinoid system and whose results mimic those of CBD. I explore the best known in this section.

Coming full circle with tree bark

Users report the same benefits from bark-derived CBD, though not much evidence or research exists as to its effectiveness. Its only reported usage I have uncovered was in the form of edibles from Grön, a confectionary out of Portland, Oregon. Grön was the first (and only, as of this writing) company documented to use a noncannabis-derived CBD at its inception. Currently they are using hemp.

Note: This form of CBD actually touches a bit of gray area as to whether it qualifies as naturally derived or synthesized. As it was historically indicated by the company, it's naturally derived *and* synthesized. They were quoted as saying "Our CBD is created through a natural product assembly which involves combining the evergreen with citrus under heat and pressure."

Focusing on the flowers

The phytocannabinoid chemicals found in cannabis are also produced by other plants and flowers; some plants produce cannabimimetics. You may already familiar with many of these plants as superfoods.

>> **Sunflowers:** Cannabinoid-like compounds that mimic cannabigerol (CBG) are present in a unique genus of sunflower called *Helichrysum*. This sunflower also contains amorfrutins, which reduce blood sugar and have anti-inflammatory effects much like CBD.

>> **Echinacea:** Echinacea, also known as coneflower, is full of cannabimimetics. Echinacea interacts with the brain receptor that regulates the immune function of inflammation, among other things. This plant is used in the treatment of conditions from arthritis to colds and migraines.

>> **Electric daisy:** The electric daisy is also known as the "toothache plant." It contains a cannabimimetic (N-isobutylamides) that can block pain receptors at nerve endings and thus is powerful for treating toothaches.

>> **Chinese rhododendron:** Folic acids in this flower act like cannabinoids by helping with inflammatory and pain response. Cannabinoid-like derivatives help reduce muscle contractions.

Exploring other similar compounds

Beyond flowers, a host of other plant-based goodies have cannabimimetic compounds:

>> **Cacao:** Cacao is known as a joyful compound; no wonder people eat chocolate to boost a bad mood. Its active compound is anandamide, a cannabinoid native to the human body.

Anandamide has a cool linguistic origin. The word actually comes from the Sanskrit word *ananda,* which literally translates to "bliss."

>> **Black truffles:** Black truffles also contain anandamide. This "joy" molecule is supposedly what causes truffle pigs to hunt for the mushrooms so furiously.

>> **Black peppercorn:** Black pepper prevents endocannabinoid uptake and acts like a cannabinoid in the body. It has been known to have anti-inflammatory properties, much like other cannabinoid compounds. Also containing the terpene beta-caryophyllene, black pepper compounds cannabis-like effects. (The earlier section "Exploring terpenes and flavonoids" has details on terpenes; you can find out which types of hemp strains contain beta-caryophyllene in "Investigating the Hemp Strains and Varieties.")

>> **Kava:** Kava has incredible calming effects and may even relieve anxiety and chronic pain. It contains compounds called *kavalactones;* one of them interacts directly with the brain receptors that help regulate pain.

Choosing between Synthetic and Natural CBD

The debate over getting CBD naturally or synthesizing it is in full swing, and both options have their merits. *Synthesizing,* in this case, means creating a man-made version of CBD. (The scientific term for it is *biomimicry.*) Companies are already hard at work creating their own versions of CBD synthetically. The ultimate goal is mass production for the consumer market.

The main argument for the synthetic process is the cost benefits that come from efficient production. Early studies show that CBD can in fact be created in a lab. Additionally, synthetic CBD looks like a viable option as over-the-counter and pharmaceutical markets around cannabis develop.

Another issue is the THC problem. Early tests have shown that naturally derived CBD can be converted to THC with simple lab procedures. THC is a psychedelic and, as of this writing, illegal substance that requires control at the federal level. The concern is that science-savvy criminals could easily convert the natural CBD in drugs to the illegal THC for profit. The black market and drug abuse (largely of opiates) are already huge problems, so the concern is legitimate. Synthetic CBD, on the other hand, cannot be converted to THC in a lab and therefore prevents the potential for entry into the illicit market.

Proponents of natural CBD point to the environmental implications. The considerate farming and growth of the hemp industry for CBD production creates jobs as well as natural healing medicine. Besides, the byproducts and positive implications of hemp growing are vast: carbon offsets, soil remediation, fiber production, and more.

One of the largest current arguments for natural CBD is the entourage effect I discuss in "Debating the benefits of using the whole plant versus the sum of its parts" earlier in the chapter. If using all parts of the plant brings the most benefits, how can lab-created CBD compare?

The counterargument from the scientific community is that the variables of nature prevent the kind of scaling up needed for mass production. Science wants to repeat results for control of effectiveness. But strain and varietal variation mean that no two plants are going to present the same chemical features, at least not long-term. That makes replicating medicinal compounds and results on use and application impossible.

Chapter **3**

Looking into What CBD Does

You know the old saying: When life gives you CBD, make pillows and lozenges and. . . . At least, that seems to be the philosophy of the CBD market, which has been absolutely inundated with product. But what CBD is and how it works can be confusing for the novice consumer.

I use this chapter as a way to unpack the available science around CBD. I discuss not just the scientific nature of the molecule but also the theoretical applications. The information here can be quite helpful in developing a plan to use CBD in a way that works best for your mind and body.

Discovering What Makes CBD Work

The diversity of interactions CBD is capable of can address imbalances in your body, thus creating *homeostasis*, or balance in the body's system. The next sections explain how CBD works in your body and compares that chemical to THC.

Comparing and contrasting CBD and THC

As I discuss in Chapter 2, *cannabinoids* are a class of plant chemicals found in the cannabis plant that parallel your body's own *endocannabinoids* — your internal human cannabinoids. Cannabidiol (CBD) is one of many cannabinoids in any cannabis plant.

REMEMBER

Cannabis is a broad umbrella term that may refer to up to three different plant types. *Cannabis sativa, Cannabis indica,* and *Cannabis ruderalis* are all flowering plants that are informally just called cannabis. (Hemp, also known as industrial hemp, is a nonpsychoactive variety of the *Cannabis sativa L.* plant.)

What makes each of the varieties of cannabis similar, and historically prohibited, is that each contains a chemical compound known as tetrahydrocannabinol (THC). *THC* is the psychoactive compound in cannabis; it's the compound that gives you a "high" (scientifically referred to as the "psychedelic experience").

TECHNICAL STUFF

Almost the entire cannabis plant, from leaves to stalks to flowers and stems, contains CBD. However, the largest concentrations of cannabinoids are in the resins on the flowers of a cannabis plant. Common cannabis mythology suggests that hemp doesn't bud and flower like other cannabis grown specifically for its THC and psychedelic properties. But more and more hemp is coming to full flower and being sold as CBD cannabis with variable amounts of THC — some as low as 0.3 percent, making it legally qualify as hemp in the United States.

CBD and THC have the same molecular formula (2 oxygen molecules, 30 hydrogen molecules, and 21 carbon molecules, if you're interested). Despite their identical molecular composition, CBD and THC are different in several important ways:

>> **Their atomic arrangements are unique.**

>> **CBD and THC interact with your body's endocannabinoid system in very distinct ways that can affect your mood and physiology.** For example, many people use CBD as an anti-anxiety treatment, while some studies have found that high concentrations of THC can increase anxious feelings.

>> **Legally speaking, THC is a controlled substance and CBD isn't.**

>> **CBD is more largely decriminalized.** Nearly every U.S. state allows CBD products to be sold, with some inherent rules and regulations. But fewer than a dozen states have legalized the recreational use of THC-dominant products.

Seeing how CBD interacts with the endocannabinoid system

The *endocannabinoid system (ECS)* is the most important system in the human body related to the benefits and interactions of cannabis and CBD. Your ECS has two receptors designed to receive and positively interact with CBD. In more complex interactions, CBD actually triggers your body to produce more of its own endocannabinoids.

TECHNICAL STUFF

The term *endocannabinoid* refers to the internal cannabinoid, coming from the Latin term *endo,* which means "internal." Scientists actually named this system after the cannabinoid system from the cannabis plant.

REMEMBER

As of this writing, none of the research shows whether one form of CBD is better than another for treating particular conditions. So scientists don't yet know whether CBD contained in a whole-plant hemp extract or isolated CBD in carrier oil is more effective. How the different forms of CBD interact with the cannabinoid and other receptors in the human body, and how CBD modifies these systems for better or worse, is also yet to be researched.

The following sections detail how CBD molecules interact with receptors in your brain and beyond.

Blocking THC from receptors

Receptors are proteins that bind to neurotransmitter molecules to create a signal that tells your body to perform a particular function. This binding and linking is like a lock-and-key system that unlocks a series of events. For example, the way that CBD attaches itself to receptors is a key that can unlock (that is, cause or accelerate) a reaction that addresses imbalances and promotes equilibrium.

These receptors exist all over the human body, from the brain to every internal organ. You have a host of receptors in your body — in your skin and throughout your organs — that interact with CBD, which makes you a great candidate for supplementing with CBD. (Unless you aren't a human, in which case the research is still out for you.)

The ECS is composed of two notable receptors: the cannabinoid receptor 1 (CB1, found in the brain and nervous system) and cannabinoid receptor 2 (CB2, found throughout the immune and other operating systems). These receptors are designed to receive information through cannabinoid chemicals. The body naturally produces these cannabinoids, and they're also delivered through foods and nutrients. CBD has been shown to interact with the receptor system by interfering with other cannabinoids' ability to directly bind to the receptors. Imagine a game of billiards. The pockets are the receptors; the solid balls are CBD, and the striped balls are another cannabinoid — for example, THC. The striped ball's (THC's) goal is to get into (bind with) the pocket (receptor). If a solid ball (CBD) stops just in front of the pocket, it's technically interacting with the pocket by preventing the striped ball from going in.

REMEMBER

The evidence doesn't actually suggest that CBD and THC are in opposition (as balls in the billiards example are). Some theories that suggest they're actually complementary; plant medicine history lends itself to those theories because every strain and variety of the cannabis plant has both CBD and THC in some concentration.

TALKING ABOUT CLINICAL ENDOCANNABINOID DEFICIENCY

It's no big secret that our human systems are chock full of deficiencies, mostly nutritional. So you probably won't be surprised when I tell you that we have an endocannabinoid deficiency, too (officially called *clinical endocannabinoid deficiency,* or *CED*). This piece of endocannabinoid science is in its theoretical state, much like all cannabinoid and endocannabinoid research.

Endocannabinoid deficiency shows up when your body's endocannabinoid system is operating in a state of malfunction. Researchers don't know what could lead to a deficiency in the endocannabinoid system, so they've been exploring whether a variety of treatment-resistant syndromes may result from CED. Potential issues linked to CED include fibromyalgia, migraines, chronic fatigue, and irritable bowel syndrome (IBS). Not stuff you want to ignore, even if your body would let you.

Whether CED is the cause of migraines and various other treatment-resistant syndromes is still unclear. What is clear is that a more balanced system can help reduce symptoms from these conditions. Your endocannabinoid system loves balance; this concept of balance is called *endocannabinoid tone.*

So what, outside of your own bodily capability of producing cannabinoids, can help you meet this deficiency? You can incorporate a few helpful ingredients — such as chocolate (cacao), black pepper, and rosemary — into your diet. And of course, there's cannabis. The puzzle piece that fits like no other. (Simply or exclusively supplementing with cannabinoids such as CBD may or may not address endocannabinoid tone. No one knows yet.)

(**Note:** Don't go searching the internet to see whether you suffer from "clinical endocannabinoid deficiency." It's just as new as all other cannabis science, and it's far less supported than other long-standing theories about deficiencies and treatments in Western medicine.)

This blocking is significant because if THC cannabinoids directly bind to the CB1 and CB2 receptors, you get a psychedelic effect. CBD prevents this "high" sensation. This changed interaction isn't good or bad; it's just part of a process.

Interestingly, CBD's interaction with those receptors can increase the body's endocannabinoid production by preventing the enzymes that break down endocannabinoids from doing their jobs. In your body, increased endocannabinoid production can potentially be beneficial (see the nearby sidebar for more information).

Checking out other receptors

CB1 and CB2 aren't the only receptors in town. CBD has the incredible capability of interacting with more than 72 different receptors in the human body. Luckily, CBD's promiscuity lends it to diverse applications, interactions, and functions. (Check out the preceding section for more on CBD's interaction with CB1 and CB2).

Some of these other receptors and their functions are

>> **TRPV1 receptors:** CBD binds to this transitory receptor known for temperature regulation. It's also recognized for mediating pain response and perception.

>> **GABA-A receptor:** GABA-A binds to neurons to decrease their activity; essentially, it calms them from overactivity that results in fear and anxiety. CBD is shown to change the shape of this receptor, increasing its calming effects on the brain. Preliminary research suggests it may go so far as to act as a sedative.

>> **Serotonin:** Serotonin is a neurotransmitter that can directly affect your mood and emotions. When CBD interacts with TRPV1, it in turn can activate serotonin, reducing anxiety and boosting mood while mitigating pain response. Plainly speaking, CBD may relieve chronic anxiety.

>> **Mu opioid receptors:** Mu receptors are one of many different types of opioid receptors on nerve cells. They primarily determine how strong of a pain-relieving effect an opioid has. CBD interacts with mu opioid receptors in a way that potentially amplifies the effects of opioids. In other words, CBD may enhance the pain-relieving properties of opioids like morphine.

>> **Dopamine:** The dopamine molecule is a feel-good neurotransmitter. It plays a key role in human behavior, affecting goal-directed behavior and learning. CBD increases the quantity of dopamine in your body.

Recognizing CBD's Physical and Mental Effects

Dr. Bradley Alger, one of the most recognized researchers in the endocannabinoid brain sciences, notes that "the endocannabinoids are literally a bridge between body and mind. By understanding the endocannabinoid system, we begin to see a mechanism that could connect brain activity and states of physical health and disease."

The true nature of CBD and how it can work with the human body is still somewhat unknown (thanks, lack of research), but some of the most affected conditions are seeing some relief with CBD.

REMEMBER

How you feel after ingesting CBD may be wildly different from how someone else feels. This difference is even more likely if the CBD is balancing your ECS, because an imbalanced ESC will likely make other parts of your body feel a bit askew. Because of the degree of variability, I outline the typical effects on CBD in various conditions here; I dive into these conditions and CBD's effects on them in greater detail in Part 3 of this book.

CBD is a jack of all trades. Researchers hail it as an anti-inflammatory, antioxidant, *neuroprotective* (a fancy word meaning it protects your brain's neurons), antipsychotic, antimicrobial, and pain reliever.

>> For reasons ranging from diet to genetics, inflammation is a common human complaint. CBD acts as an anti-inflammatory and antioxidant — ramping up the body's defense system. Oxidation and deterioration are a natural part of

the slowing of cell regeneration. CBD has been linked to hampering those effects. It also treats irritation, redness, and bruising.

>> CBD is hailed as an antipsychotic, regulating mood, thinking, and perception as it interacts with the receptors in the brain. As a neuroprotective, it reduces toxicity from external factors.

>> In research around *neurodegenerative* disorders such as Huntington's disease and Alzheimer's disease, the way CBD blocks and disrupts the binding of the molecules that contribute to negative effects may have positive impacts.

>> In topical circumstances, CBD can fight against bacteria.

>> Pain management may be one of the most exciting discoveries to date because more than one-third of the U.S. population deals with pain. The limitless applications of CBD as a pain reliever dominate the current research trend.

>> CBD contributes to increased relaxation by decreasing tension and muscle stress. Better sleep, deeper rest, and diminished anxiety are being reported across a variety of CBD users.

>> Overall, CBD seems to balance bodily systems, including mood and digestion.

>> In the skincare realm, increased moisture retention is a lovely effect many users enjoy.

Chapter **4**

Extracting, Infusing, and Producing CBD

The hemp cannabis plant in and of itself is valuable for many purposes. It has been providing powerful and positive experiences for humans for centuries. But its rock-star component, CBD, can be tough to isolate. CBD has many versatile uses, but to get a usable concentration of it, you have to extract, isolate, distill, or infuse it. (Well, not you personally, necessarily, but someone does.)

Extraction is the process of separating the plant matter from the other chemical parts. You can essentially consume the plant in its whole form and get good results for many conditions, and in some scenarios, that's the ideal method of consumption. However, many Americans' interactions with cannabis center on byproducts. I want to familiarize you with different forms of CBD you may encounter more readily, so in this chapter, I explore the different methods of extracting CBD.

Familiarizing Yourself with Extraction Methods

Extraction likely existed long before humans had a way to record how they did it and why. Over time, the processes have evolved. CBD extraction methods have become more advanced and refined in the same way that human devices for light shifted from campfires to candles to lightbulbs. Some of the methods for home use pale in comparison to the complexities used in commercial settings. On the other hand, some commercial applications still utilize traditional methods because of the outcome.

Different methods have different effects on the end product. Some methods are better known for leaving residue, scent, or taste. Some have a negative environmental impact, and all have wildly different cost implications.

REMEMBER

Knowing a bit about the extraction process is imperative in understanding the value of a particular product for your particular needs. CBD is part of a fairly new commercial industry. The formulators, extractors, growers, and so forth that create commercial products rely on their personal judgment. They work with the method that's best for them, now, in the developmental stages of their businesses and the industry. Those methods may not be the best method for that product or your body. Make sure you know the what, why, and how of what you're consuming.

Solvent extraction is the most common method in current use. Here's a quick list of solvents used in extractions:

>> Alcohol

>> Ethanol

>> Ether

>> Butane

>> Propane

>> Carbon dioxide (CO_2)

>> Double CO_2

>> Oil

These solvents essentially dissolve the plant matter, and then the remaining matter gets removed through a mesh sieve or something similar. The solvent is then heated to the point of evaporation, leaving behind only the plant extracts. Some of these forms of extraction involve heat, time and pressure, as there are variations to the process of extraction with each solvent.

The challenges associated with the solvents are directly related to the fact that the extraction methods often leave byproducts. For example, butane is itself a byproduct extracted in the production of crude oil. Even if all the butane is removed in the CBD extraction process, some residuals from the production of the butane may still be left over. As the industry evolves, safer methods will follow. A favorite of the higher volume extraction facilities is Double C02 Extraction. That term will appear on multitudes of labels. It is also favored for being one of the cleaner forms of large-volume extraction. Alcohol and oil solvent extractions remain among the favorites for ease and efficacy for many extractors, and for now, I tend to be partial to these two all-natural food-safe extraction forms.

Discerning the Qualities of Kinds of Extractions

Familiarizing yourself with the different types of extractions, and the products they yield, is important. This section sets you on the journey of becoming an informed and scientifically savvy CBD consumer.

>> **Full-spectrum CBD:** *Full-spectrum CBD* is the first outcome of any extraction. It carries all the parts of the plant leaves, the fiber, and the plant matter itself. The predominant theories are that full-spectrum is the most therapeutic of the extracts. Processing it to remove extra compounds results in the forms that follow.

>> **Broad-spectrum CBD:** As I write this, a lot of CBD products on the market have broad-spectrum oil as an active ingredient. A *broad-spectrum extract* is a result of removing one or more of the chemical compounds found in a full-spectrum extract (see the preceding section). A compound often targeted for removal is THC because, from a legal standpoint, CBD products are required to have no more than 0.3 percent THC.

>> **Distillate:** *Distillation* is a further step in processing and creating an extract without taste or aroma. Some call it a purification process. In a world with so many added chemicals, having a short ingredient list has become a selling point. Distillate is made to maintain a specific cannabinoid (such as THC) and nothing else, creating the desired potency without the effects of other components. (*Cannabinoids* are the plant chemicals specific to cannabis and hemp plants; you can read more about them in Chapter 2.)

>> **Isolate:** *Isolate* is exactly that: an isolated chemical compound. In the case of CBD, an isolate is solely the cannabinoid CBD without any other terpenes, flavonoids, or cannabinoids. (I cover these substances in more detail in Chapter 2.) Isolate is your classic catch-22: It's adored for its simplicity and equally unappreciated for its lack of complexity.

>> **Other forms:** Other forms of CBD aren't directly derived from extraction but instead are yielded from further processing of an extracted form of CBD, full-spectrum, broad-spectrum, distillate and Isolate. For example, *nanopartializing* CBD is the process of making the chemical itself smaller. *Water-soluble* CBD is the result of suspending oil-based CBD into a water-based compound with an emulsion that keeps the two repelling agents, water and oil, from separating. These forms are popular because they're believed to make the CBD easier for the body to take in, but the evidence on them is insufficient.

Identifying the Forms Resulting from Extraction

The incredible diversity of form is what makes the secondary market for CBD and other cannabis products so interesting. You can find some of the most common forms in the following sections.

The CBD market continues to evolve. By the time this book publishes, some other form may well be all the rage.

CBD RSO

RSO stands for Rick Simpson Oil. Often considered a grandfather of the cannabis movement, Simpson was known for his forward-thinking, alternative approach to treating cancer with highly concentrated cannabis. This full-spectrum oil, also called Phoenix Tears, uses the whole plant except the fiber. It has a honey-like consistency and is very dark amber or brown. Though RSO is more common in the medicinal cannabis market with THC as a component, more and more versions with CBD flower extractions are starting to appear.

Consumption method varies by patient. The recommended approach involves small doses from a needleless syringe contraption. Some people prefer to take it under the tongue *(sublingually)*, while others put a little dab on a piece of food.

CBD distillate

Butane and alcohol extractions remain some of the most common with distillate, largely because of the consumption methods that follow. By extracting the CBD molecule along with other plant chemicals and plant matter, producers begin to form a refined version of the plant, *distillate*. It morphs from a sticky paste to an oil, depending on the distillation agent and the amount of time. Some prefer this method because it's less expensive. As long as legality and price point dominate the market, it's here to stay. For CBD in particular, distillation is a necessary step for removing THC to meet legal regulations.

Adding CBD distillate to a base of carrier oil or alcohol creates a host of ways to use it, from as an ingredient in a topical to as a topical in its own right to ingestible and more! For example, a popular use involves adding CBD distillate to carrier oils such as hemp seed oil, MCT oil, or the like for sublingual use or for vaporizing. Many people prefer inhalation via smoking as a dab, wax, resin, rosin, and more. I break down the aforementioned forms of consumption in Chapter 7.

CBD isolate

Isolate is a pure CBD chemical extract with no other compounds from the plant or extraction method. Perfect extraction creates a clear, whitish, crystalline form that can become a white powder if crushed. Isolate that isn't highly refined often has a damp, yellowish appearance, a reflection of its origin.

You can cleanly add isolate to a carrier oil, leaving no residual cannabis taste or smell. It's mostly still used as an additive; however, people have been known to vaporize it exclusively for its effects.

Infusing CBD

Infusion is a common DIY method of extracting the beneficial compounds from plant matter's chemicals and aromas. The process is worth exploring more if you have the time and interest.

Discovering the basics of CBD infusions

Most of cannabis's plant matter is in lipid form, so the best way to create an infusion is with another oil-based material — butter, coconut oil, ghee (a clarified butter), or whatever. This combination results in *bioavailability*, or your body's ability to take in the chemicals. Soaking the plant matter for an extended period imparts the valuable chemicals and aromas are into the carrier or base oil. Heat can also create this transfer as long as the heat isn't so high that it compromises the plant's integrity.

You can use CBD flower to supplement almost anything. It's a great addition in butter for cookies, ghee for curries, oils for salad dressing, and so on. You do want to know the actual concentration of full-spectrum plant chemicals you're infusing into your oil. *All* reputable providers — at the dispensary or online — will provide you with the certificate of analysis (COA), which outlines the concentration of cannabinoids and sometimes even terpenes in what you're buying. The CBD concentration is written as a percentage; common numbers range from 5 percent to 25 percent, with 5 being low strength and 25 being the highest.

TIP

You can also figure out concentrations yourself, as I explain in the following section.

Calculating concentrations like a champ

To calculate CBD concentrations, you have to convert the percentage of CBD in the flower to the number of milligrams in the volume of the flower. From there, you separate the volume into milligram servings based on your dosing requirements; that may be anywhere from five to a couple of hundred milligrams depending on your needs.

Don't worry; you don't need some fancy graphing calculator to figure this stuff out. The app on your phone is just fine. Here's an example.

You have 1 gram of 15 percent CBD flower, and you want a 10-milligram dose per 1 tablespoon of oil. Convert 15 percent to a decimal (divide 15 by 100) to get 0.15.

Convert 1 gram to milligrams; 1 gram is 1,000 milligrams. Multiply 0.15 by 1,000 to get the amount of CBD per gram of flower.

0.15 CBD × 1,000 milligrams = 150 milligrams/1 gram of flower

For a 10-milligram dose, divide 150 by 10 to get the number of servings.

150 milligrams CBD/10 milligrams CBD = 15 servings

Therefore, you need 15 tablespoons of oil for 1 gram of flower to have a 10 milligram/1 tablespoon ratio of CBD to oil.

Two grams of the same flower would be 300 milligrams per gram of flower (2 × 150 = 300), 3 grams would be 450 milligrams, and so on.

TIP

If you decide to infuse butter and bake with it, the same math applies.

Infusing CBD at home

The best way to pick up a new skill is to do it. Because infusions are so time-tested and safe to make and use, now is a great time to dive in. You'll need a few items that may already be lying around your kitchen if you delight in trying out new or specialty recipes. To be fully prepared to begin, grab a grinder or mortar and pestle, something to cook the infusion in (more on that in Step 3), and a fine mesh strainer. Cheesecloth also works!

1. **Figure out the concentration.**

   I explain the math for this process in the preceding section.

2. **Grind the flower.**

   Grinding the flower makes exposing every little bit and immersing it in your oil of choice easier.

3. **Combine the base oil or fat in the appropriate volume to the cooker.**

   Olive oil, coconut oil, butter, ghee, sesame oil — the options are endless from an oil standpoint.

   As for the cooking device, you want something that controls the heat over time so you get a proper infusion. A host of tools are readily available, from stovetop double boilers to slow cookers. You can also get options made specifically for the cannabis and hemp market. Levo and Ardent are two great brands.

4. **Cover the cooker, set it to high, and cook for one hour.**

5. **Turn the cooker down to low and cook for two to three hours.**

   The slow and low heat is important here because the heat and time create a chemical reaction necessary to activate the cannabinoids in the CBD flower. This reaction is properly known as *decarboxylation.*

6. **Strain the mixture through a fine mesh strainer or a cheesecloth to remove the plant matter.**

7. **Store your infused oil in an airtight container.**

   An airtight container is important here because when you expose cannabis to oxygen over a long period, it activates prematurely. That early activation ultimately degrades the potency and flavor. If you use butter or animal fat, put it in the fridge or freezer if you don't intend to use it all right away.

Using CBD Extracts to Make a Product

Whether you make CBD extract at home or you buy one of the many available in stores, making, cooking, or preparing CBD anything at home is easy breezy. It's as simple as having another ingredient to add to whatever you're making, as long as what you're making requires some sort of fatty or oil-based substance.

Creating a useable topical or consumable product

Creating an effective home product by using CBD is quite simple if you stick to fatty oil and animal fat extracts. (You can use extracts that have other compounds in them or that aren't fat-soluble, but that's outside the scope of this book.) The most important piece is knowing how to create proper doses within your recipe. The formulas are pretty straightforward:

> Amount of CBD in container (in milligrams)/Size of dose (in milligrams) = Number of CBD doses per container

> Volume of vial for your final product (in milliliters)/Number of CBD doses = Volume of product dose

Here's an example: Say you have a 315-milligram tincture vial of CBD, and your personal dose is 15 milligrams. Plug those numbers into the formula, and you find that you can get 21 doses from that vial:

> 315 milligrams/15 milligrams = 21 doses

Now look at the size of the vial for the infused product you're creating. Divide that by the number of doses (21) to get the size of your product dose (basically, one serving size of your infused product):

> 30 milliliters/21 doses = 1.43 milliliters/dose

For this example, 1.43 milliliters of your infused product will give you the 15-milligram dose of CBD you're looking for.

REMEMBER

Like almost any other plant matter, CBD extracts and products have an expiration date, so be sure to store your goodies properly in an airtight container. If you use butter or animal fat, put it in the fridge or freezer if you don't intend to use it all right away.

Including complementary substances

To get the most out of your CBD, invite some other ingredients to the party! Technically, whatever base you use is the first complementary substance in any home-made CBD product because it's a complement to the lipid-based CBD chemical that needs a carrier. But you can also add other compounds or ingredients that may enhance CBD's effects. This list is endless, and it starts with a whole host of other plants that contain similar plant chemicals to cannabis, like terpenes, from linalool to myrcene. (Flip to Chapter 2 for more on terpenes.) It also means vitamins like B, C, and E, found in oils and minerals like sodium, and magnesium found in salts and Epsom salts.

For example, the best-recognized properties of CBD are its anti-inflammatory effects. To double down on those benefits, pair CBD with other anti-inflammatories. Natural anti-inflammatory plants include arnica, turmeric, and black pepper (just to name a few). These options are great additions for any topical. (Actually, you can use turmeric both topically and internally.)

Two other famous benefits of CBD are the improvement of sleep and stress relief. Melatonin, found in tart cherries and goji berries as well as chamomile and jasmine (among many more), may assist with sleep. Lemon and other citrus fruits, peppermint, and lavender are popular, effective solutions for stress and anxiety. Combine any one of these ingredients with hemp flower in a nice tea.

REMEMBER

CBD can only do so much, and it varies by individual and dose. An incredible diversity of other supplements and nutrients help support specific body systems, and understanding what your body needs so you can address that specifically is important.

Chapter 5

Doing the Math: The Pluses and Minuses of CBD

You've picked up a book on CBD. You're curious; maybe you have a condition that has been hard to treat, or you have symptoms from a chronic condition and aren't happy with the current options. That feeling is totally understandable, and you're completely right to pursue something a little off the beaten track if you aren't finding the relief you need.

Surprise: This chapter looks at some general pros and cons regarding CBD use. There's no shortage of chatter about the potential benefits of CBD, but proving beyond a shadow of a doubt that CBD does what marketers and brands say it does has been hard. Supposed benefits include relief from fibromyalgia, advanced arthritis, sleeplessness, fatigue, GI conditions, neuropathic conditions, topical inflammation, and chronic pain, among others. But the information available is basically some rudimentary science and some serious compilations of anecdotal/experiential evidence, so no one can say with 100 percent certainty CBD does any one thing. It *is* largely recognized by scientists, researchers, and users alike to alleviate symptoms of inflammation, which is a component of tons of conditions, including the ones I just mentioned.

Beyond the sheer volume of misinformation that's out there, a few actual negatives of CBD use have cropped up. This chapter helps you examine which claims are legitimate.

Realizing the Potential Benefits: The Four Pillars of CBD (and an Added Bonus)

This section explores the four most significant pillars of CBD care cases to date. These pillars are the most common ailments plaguing the American population today. Additionally, we explore the topic of CBD skincare and beauty, and while it is just as much a pillar to some, it is not as important to others. Among *the others* are the regulating bodies that impose guidelines on product claims and marketing.

REMEMBER

To be clear out of the gates, I need to define *relief.* According to Merriam-Webster, it's the "removal or lightening of something oppressive, painful, or distressing." Terms such as *cure, fix, remedy,* and the like represent direct medical claims. In the United States, only items with FDA approval can make such claims. So I talk about CBD in terms of relief but always precede claims with a conditional word like "may" or "potentially." Always remember that CBD is not a cure; it's a hypothetical remedy that can vary in effectiveness based its application and the condition being aided.

Relieving stress and anxiety

For the sake of eliminating confusion between stress and anxiety, I break them down separately here. *Stress* is a natural response to help address circumstances that require a level of heightened mental alertness and physical response. *Anxiety* is a reaction to stress. Anxiety is painfully persistent even when the triggers aren't present.

TIP

I look at stress and anxiety in comic book terms. Think about stress as Spider-Man's Spidey sense, which alerts him of impending danger. Now imagine that Spider-Man routinely feels his Spidey sense even in nonthreatening circumstances, with no underlying cause. That's anxiety.

Stress experiences are caused by mental and physical situations that result in symptoms such as pain, sleeplessness, gastrointestinal (GI) issues, anger, frustration, skin issues (which I discuss later in the chapter), and general fatigue. The body reacts to stress by releasing stress hormones, including cortisol and adrenaline, that push the body into a state of emergency action. In this state, your body is basically in overdrive — pumping blood more quickly through your system, increasing your heart rate, tightening your muscles, heightening your senses, and so on. The most identifiable feelings of stress manifest as nervousness, exhausting thoughts, lack of focus, compromised judgment, and disorganization.

Constantly living in this stress state has been associated with a multitude of overall health problems, even heart attacks and death. Early studies have shown that CBD modifies the body's chemical interaction with cortisol in a sedative way. It mitigates stress by preventing the overflow of cortisol.

Though anxiety can feel much like stress, it's actually clinically diagnosable. Because CBD seems to be apt at relieving stress responses, it also seems to be beneficial in cases of anxiety.

Soothing mood conditions

Your mood is affected by so many things, from outside stressors to chemical imbalances in the body. CBD can be helpful for clinical conditions (such as psychosis, clinical depression, and PTSD) and nonclinical conditions (such as sadness, feelings of isolation, frustration, and more) because it "calms" the brain by supporting the hippocampus. The *hippocampus* is the area of the brain responsible for behavior, among other functions.

CBD has been associated with relieving depression and improving your mood, and it has been indicated in studies to have antidepressant effects.

Helping manage sleep issues

Sleep conditions, from insomnia to sleep apnea and narcolepsy, are an epidemic. According to the American Sleep Association (sleepassociation.org), such conditions affect between 50 and 70 million Americans, and more than 70 percent of the adult population reports insufficient sleep.

Sleep studies in their early phases are indicating incredible results with measured doses of CBD. They suggest doses around 25 milligrams can help patients fall asleep, and then varying doses ranging from 50 to 160 milligrams can help people stay asleep. The studies indicate potential applications effective for the treatment of *insomnia,* a sleep condition that results in consistent feelings of unrest. And as I note in the preceding section, CBD seems to interrupt the body's cortisol secretion, creating sedative effects that can also help with sleep issues.

Some studies have indicated that alertness is an effect of CBD use, and while some are taking it specifically to improve alertness, some take CBD to sleep. If taking CBD creates a sensation of sleep difficulty, exploring conditions and the root cause of sleeplessness are most certainly in order.

Relieving pain and physical ailments

Promising research indicates that CBD can reduce inflammation and chronic pain, which is one of the contributors to the opioid epidemic. Additionally, patients are unlikely to build up a tolerance to CBD; that means they don't have to increase dosages to maintain effects (another issue with opioids).

CBD affects a variety of enzymes throughout the body, including in the skin. For example, it suppresses the production of TNF-a, a pro-inflammatory enzyme found throughout the body, including the skin. CBD also promotes two receptors responsible for anti-inflammatory effects: TRPV-1, or *vanilloid*, and PPAR-y, or *gamma*.

A doctor once told me in passing at a conference that CBD is already known to interact with over 76 different receptors in the body. Whoa!

The vanilloid receptor itself is responsible for decreasing the intensity of pain signals and the overall nervous system's response to pain. Acute pain is caused by physical trauma of some sort, whether it has a known cause (like a shin bang or broken bone) or unknown cause (like a migraine or backache). For surface-level acute pain, you can use topical CBD treatments; for more severe acute pain, particularly internal, ingestible CBD is a better choice. Regardless of the pain type, you want to choose a CBD medium with a rapid onset so you don't have to wait around for relief.

Transdermal patches are starting to fill that gap in the topical space because they offer internal relief with a topical treatment (head to Chapter 1 for more on transdermal treatment). Otherwise, the fastest onset is inhalation or *sublingual* (under the tongue) tinctures. Doses for pain should be higher than supplemental doses, and you can use them until the pain is alleviated without worrying about becoming dependent.

Chronic physical pain can sometimes have a neurological component when the pain has persisted over a long time and may have a historical association with psychological or physiological trauma. The nerves can signal pain even when no physical reason for it actually exists. Theories and early studies indicate that a controlled amount of THC is the most significant relief opportunity in cannabis for this kind of pain. The current legal limit for THC in full-spectrum CBD is 0.3 percent, which just may not be enough for that kind of pain experience. But everybody is different, and giving CBD a try for such pain may still help. High doses of full-spectrum CBD and maybe even broad-spectrum or isolate may work for some because inflammation is often still at the core of many pain problems. (Chapter 4 has details on full- and broad-spectrum CBD and isolate.)

TIP

Arthritis patients are seeing deeper relief with topical applications. With the overwhelming lack of scientific studies and clinical trials available, people who are experiencing a lack of relief from traditional options are trying CBD as a remedy and finding results. The Arthritis Foundation conducted a poll of its community and discovered that 29 percent currently use CBD in a liquid or topical form and reported improvement in physical pain, stiffness, and function.

Promoting skin health and beauty

Inflammation is one of the largest contributors to skin stress or conditions, so CBD is showing promise in topical applications for the treatment of conditions like eczema, acne, psoriasis, and dryness. Early studies and a new clinical trial are indicating that synthetic CBD specifically is proving beneficial in the treatment of acne. (You can read more about synthetic CBD in Chapter 2.) The antifungal and antimicrobial properties of CBD also lend themselves to addressing skin concerns.

CBD isn't believed to bond with the *endocannabinoid* receptors in the ECS system (which involves your body's internal human *cannabinoids,* chemicals in hemp and cannabis). It does interact with the receptors, and a whole host of other receptors, including the vanilloid and gamma receptors I discuss in the earlier section "Relieving pain and physical ailments." The vanilloid receptor is responsible for balance *(homeostasis)* in the skin. The gamma receptor is responsible for cell regulation, including inflammation relief.

STARTING WITHIN TO ADDRESS ROOT CAUSES

Westernized individuals often have the urge to hide or suppress symptoms, which only perpetuates the larger disease or issue. For anyone looking to topical CBD for skin relief from external stressors, I suggest turning inward first. Think about the potential internal and psychological root causes. For example, if you break out in hives each time your judgmental in-laws come to visit, perhaps that isn't a coincidence. Try to accurately identify your stressors and then use the topicals as a secondary point of skin relief.

Looking at the Pros and Cons of Supplementing with CBD

CBD is to homeopathic supplements what Madonna was to the '80s: It's just hit after hit with widespread groups of people. The diverse nature of CBD, and the considerable variety of systems within the body capable of interacting with it, makes it incredibly compatible with a wide scope of needs. Because of these chameleonlike qualities, supplementing with CBD may well be beneficial for many individuals. Supplementing not just in terms of complementing and layering with your other (compatible) treatments, but also taking it as a general support to your existing health and wellness regime to maintain a level of balance — as a preventative — potentially staving off any pending conditions.

Adjusting to daily use

Because CBD comes in so many forms and has so many uses, incorporating it into daily life can be quite simple. After all, building a routine takes only 21 days!

TIP

Try working CBD into a routine you already have going. If you drink coffee in the morning and you need a morning dose, put it in your coffee machine. If you need it at night, put it on your bedstand. If you need it a few minutes before bed, put it by your toothbrush. The options are limitless.

Personally, I've found that as a supplement, just 10 milligrams of CBD twice a day does the trick for me. I take a tincture under the tongue or add it to my morning beverage. Then I dose myself again as the early evening approaches. You can use gummies, capsules, or even snacks the same way.

REMEMBER

If you're taking CBD to relieve a condition or a symptom, you'll likely find that you notice when you don't have enough of it in your system. The reappearance of whatever your specific ailment is may be compelling enough for you to remember to take your dose or doses.

Acknowledging potential drawbacks

Every single body and operating system is different. What works for you may not work for others and in fact may really harm another person. The CBD itself isn't the only factor; you also have to consider the carrier, the packaging, the extraction process, and the consumption process. Everything matters.

WARNING

As with anything, seek the guidance of a doctor or a medicinal professional you trust to help you navigate the potential benefits and challenges. CBD is *not* for everyone. Many studies suggest that few negative side effects or incompatibility indicators exist.

That said, data is still limited. Remember to tell your doctor(s) about all the supplements, medicines, and self-medication that are part of your world, even if you don't use them regularly. As I note in the following section, CBD and other medications aren't always compatible, so doctors need to know what they're working with. Fully commit to full disclosure, even if you think that the item isn't significant enough to share or that the doctor may judge you.

Checking how CBD interacts with medication

Maybe the single most important consideration is how the body metabolizes medications. The process of breaking down your medications is an intimate part of how the medications themselves were designed to be efficient.

CBD and other cannabinoids are metabolized by various enzymes. Among those enzymes is one specifically responsible for metabolizing almost 60 percent of clinically prescribed medications. That single enzyme *can* be inhibited by CBD. When this single enzyme isn't functioning optimally, it can't break down the other medications in your body properly, potentially compromising the function of the medicines.

REMEMBER

The bottom line, the expedited or slowed metabolization of any medication, including CBD, can have unintended consequences. So, ask your doctor!

Taking responsibility for being informed

Like with anything new, you must pay attention and be responsible for anything you're introducing into your routines. Currently, CBD isn't part of a regulated market (much like supplements in general) so knowing whether you're getting what you think you are is hard. (That's why knowing what to buy, how to read labels, and so forth is important; I cover those topics in Chapter 6.)

REMEMBER

CBD is an option from the natural product marketplace. Natural products are always subject to variables — in the sun, in the soil, in the conditions in which they're grown and harvested (which can impact their chemical makeups). Acknowledging the variables in the product space makes acknowledging the variances in how different products may affect you.

If you're supplementing, you must be aware of all the other things you may encounter: reactions and side effects to just through repeated use. For instance, I have used coconut oil and *MCT oil* (a supplement made from *medium-chain triglycerides*, a type of fat) for at least ten years, on and off, in recipes. When I started supplementing with CBD, I consumed at least 1.5 milliliters of MCT oil daily for over two years. At some point, I noticed a little scratchy feeling in my throat. I had developed a minor allergy to the MCT oil, which I was able to uncover by testing CBD in other carrier oils.

Weighing the Risks and Challenges of General CBD Use

Many of the perceived risks of CBD use are based on misconceptions and misinformation (as I discuss in Chapter 1), but that doesn't mean you can discount all risks. CBD can react negatively with other medications — see the preceding sections — and even your own individual physiology. What's more, not all physicians have a deep understanding of CBD as a treatment, so getting professional guidance may take some doing. The following sections take a look at some of these factors.

REMEMBER

If the medications you're taking are vital for your basic functioning, and your doctor says CBD won't mix, it's probably a no-go for you.

Finding a doctor versed in CBD

Because legal medicinal cannabis is fairly new and not currently widespread in the United States, you may have some trouble locating a doctor knowledgeable enough to help you plan and implement your treatment. I have found that doctors tend to be more cautious if they don't have experience with cannabis as medicine.

Fortunately, with the rise of CBD and the hopeful future of cannabis legalization in the United States, you have increasing options for reaching Western and Eastern practitioners who have experience with making recommendations. Many of these resources are going to be focused on the full-spectrum, THC-containing cannabis, but a good cannabis doctor can help evaluate the benefits and risks of CBD as well. If your state allows medical cannabis, don't hesitate to get a medical cannabis card and talk to a practitioner about the implications.

TIP

Here are a couple of resources for locating a cannabis doctor:

>> HelloMD.com is a great multistate option.

>> The doctors at doctorsknox.com are internationally acclaimed and still very much focused on patient care. Their focus is on cannabinoid medicine, with expertise spanning integrative cannabinology and functional endocannabinology.

Spotting an adverse reaction to CBD

CBD does have some legitimate side effects. The most important adverse reaction to take into consideration is anything that may affect the function of your liver. Liver reactions include loss of appetite, nausea, fever, weakness, abdominal pain, vomiting, and tiredness. As noted in a study, CBD use may be a cause for concern at very high doses over 1,200 milligrams a day sustained for several weeks. The same research also reported that CBD interactions with some drugs included liver abnormalities, drowsiness, diarrhea, vomiting, and fatigue.

Users have reported other issues like dry mouth and low blood pressure that are similar to those associated with other cannabis consumption. Lightheadedness and drowsiness have also been noted.

REMEMBER

One person's goal is another person's side effect. Some people actually use CBD because of its sedative and blood-pressure-lowering qualities, but for others, those can be adverse reactions. If CBD makes you drowsy and you aren't taking it for sleep, think about the implications that may have on your functionality.

GIVING YOURSELF PERMISSION TO SEEK OTHER OPTIONS

CBD is just the tip of the cannabis iceberg. It's the most widely known and most readily accessible cannabinoid, but more than 100 cannabinoids have various benefits, from sleep to inflammation relief to antimicrobial and antibacterial properties. Beyond CBD, an incredible array of other incredible plant medicines are at your fingertips. Keep your eyes peeled, or maybe just research a little in the area of cannabinoids to see what you can find.

Search for terms such as "natural medicine" and "natural drugs," or by condition and ailment. Look for *adaptogenic botanicals,* like ginseng, ashwagandha, reishi, chaga, holy basil, and about 65 more, that counteract stressors on the body. Look for *nervines,* (plants that support the nervous system), like chamomile, lavender, and others. To make it that much easier, you can also just head straight over to my company, www.shop-poplar.com, as we have carefully crafted a marketplace to make natural medicine of all types accessible, affordable, and easy to understand.

Warning: Be wary of the "wellness" marketing that can overcomplicate and overprice some of the remedies that have been available for centuries across cultures and are available from often under-marketed brands in the United States.

2

Finding and Using CBD

Get a handle on the ins and outs of when and how to buy your CBD. Recognize how the legality of CBD varies.

Understand what products are best for your body and how to use them.

Take a look at how to use CBD safely and responsibly.

Chapter **6**

Buying CBD

N
ow that CBD is legal, you may assume that purchasing it is the easiest piece of the puzzle. But this market is a complicated industry with new rules, no regulation, and a good number of people looking to make a quick profit. Exploring all the options for making the best choices you can as an informed consumer is vital.

REMEMBER

Being a first-timer doesn't necessarily mean you're going to be making many mistakes, but it does cut you a little slack if you do.

In this chapter, I help you explore the legality of CBD from federal laws to a state-by-state basis. Because varying laws have created differences in retail and purchasing options, I cover a bit of those variables as well. Then of course there is the wonderful world of the internet, where just about anything is available at your fingertips. All of this presents a diversity of options, and with that comes the responsibility to make informed choices about who you can trust and what product is best for you. I hope to be able to distill a bit of this information for you and make it easier to make a good decision about where to buy your CBD.

Discovering What You Can Legally Buy in the United States

CBD derived from hemp is nationally legal under the 2018 Farm Bill. It's classified as an agricultural commodity, but there are lots of details and fine print. Hemp has also been removed from the Controlled Substances Act (CSA). To further complicate matters, states have taken it upon themselves to regulate CBD within their own borders, and a few have chosen to enforce stricter regulation than the national legislation requires.

This section covers what you need to know about both federal and state laws.

Following federal laws

According to the 2018 Farm Bill (also known as the Agriculture Improvement Act of 2018), hemp-derived CBD is nationally legal as long as it has less than 0.3 percent THC. Hemp meeting this condition is no longer controlled under the CSA. However, hemp-containing products that are regulated by the FDA must meet the regulating criteria of the Federal Food, Drug, and Cosmetic Act (FD&C).

REMEMBER

The FDA isn't an enforcing, regulating body of the government. However, it's the respected voice of judgment around safety in consumer-packaged goods. Cannabis, hemp, and CBD all fall under this category. In a statement, the FDA says

The FDA evaluates CBD just like any other substance we regulate, under a regulatory framework defined by law and with rigorous scientific evidence as a basis for both our regulatory approach and information we communicate. We've consistently communicated concerns and questions regarding the science, safety, and quality of many of these products based on currently available evidence. We still don't have clear answers to important questions such as what adverse reactions may be associated with CBD products and what risks are associated with the long-term use of CBD products. Better data in these areas are needed for the FDA and other public health agencies to make informed, science-based decisions that impact public health.

Being aware of the laws in your state

REMEMBER

You need to know that the legality of CBD is affected by its production. The prevalence of CBD has created an abundance of legal sources (across most states) via hemp cultivation and extraction. That said, CBD is also present in cannabis plants containing THC. Anything containing THC is heavily regulated at both the state and federal level. On a more finite level, some states regulate CBD from THC-containing cannabis plants differently based on how the substance is used. So know your state or buy from an operator you trust that knows the laws.

Dispensaries in regulated markets selling medical cannabis and adult-use cannabis often sell CBD with higher concentrations of THC. (*Adult-use* cannabis is what's commonly referred to as "recreational" cannabis.) They also sell CBD that is specifically derived from THC-rich cannabis. This type of product isn't available on a national marketplace, and state regulations don't cross borders.

The following list discusses the laws in each major region of the United States. You can also check out the map in Figure 6-1 for guidance.

>> **Early adopters:** Less than a quarter of the states are out ahead of the curve. They're passing more progressive laws around CBD than the rest of the country and cannabis legislation in general. In alphabetical order, here are the handful that allow hemp-sourced CBD, "marijuana" cannabis-sourced CBD for medical use, and "marijuana" cannabis-sourced CBD for recreational use ("marijuana" cannabis meaning THC-containing cannabis):

  - Alaska

  - California

  - Colorado

  - Illinois

  - Maine

  - Massachusetts

  - Michigan

  - Nevada

  - Oregon

  - Vermont

  - Washington

  - Washington, DC

CBD Legality Status by State
(as of May 2021)

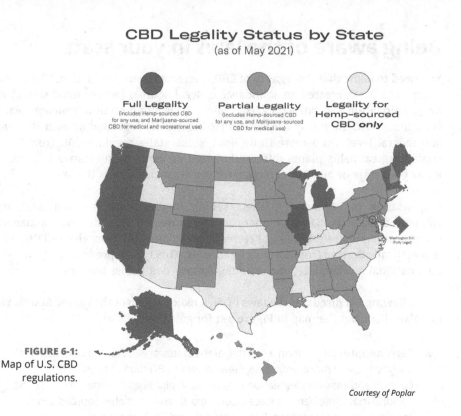

Full Legality
(includes Hemp-sourced CBD for any use, and Marijuana-sourced CBD for medical and recreational use)

Partial Legality
(includes Hemp-sourced CBD for any use, and Marijuana-sourced CBD for medical use)

Legality for Hemp-sourced CBD *only*

Washington D.C. (Fully Legal)

Courtesy of Poplar

FIGURE 6-1: Map of U.S. CBD regulations.

In these states, the CBD sourced from THC-containing plants can be sold to both adult-use (REC) and medical (MED) markets, which are both regulated dispensary outlets. CBD from hemp can be sold outside of those regulated spaces.

>> **The West Coast:** As the state that spearheaded the current pro-cannabis legislation, who better than California to be the largest force in legalizing CBD? Like its fellow coastline states Alaska and Hawaii, California makes all possible allowances for CBD access.

>> **The Northeast:** New Hampshire is the only restrictive state in the whole Northeast. All the other states in the region are on board with the federal regulations.

>> **The Southwest:** Early to the cannabis legalization community of states, this part of the world hasn't been affected by conservative state regulations around CBD. All these states follow the CBD guidelines of the Farm Bill.

>> **The rest:** The Southeast and the Midwest have the highest concentration of states with restrictions on CBD labeling, concentration, and sales outlets. These no-nonsense laws exist in South Carolina, Georgia, Mississippi, Missouri, Iowa, Nebraska, and North and South Dakota.

Promoting Medical Use

Medical use, as I define it in this book, is when CBD is specifically used as a treatment to address conditions.

Understanding the different kinds of retailers

You can access CBD in a variety of ways, and what may be best for you may not be best for another, specifically due to regulation. CBD from medical or recreational dispensaries is going to be different from what you can buy off the shelf online because of the regulations that are required for distribution in dispensaries. First and foremost, the best source is an accessible one that offers a quality product and high standards of production.

Here's a quick breakdown of the regulatory food chain:

>> **Medical dispensary:** The top of the chain is the medical dispensary. If you have access to legal cannabis in your state, you can shop at a medical dispensary. It has more-regulated (though not necessarily highest quality), forcibly transparent products available on its shelves.

>> **Adult-use dispensary:** The next level is the adult-use (sometimes called recreational) dispensary, which is also only in THC-regulated states. These sorts of dispensaries often have a greater diversity of products simply because of the larger market size for REC over the medical market.

>> **National marketplace:** The largest and most readily available marketplace is the national marketplace of hemp-derived CBD products containing less than 0.3 percent THC. These products are available across most of the United States with very few exceptions. (You can read about state CBD/THC laws in the earlier section "Being aware of the laws in your state.")

Checking quality

Labels labels labels! Any good company has detail-oriented labeling with the key information necessary to secure a sale and build both confidence and consumer trust. The following sections highlight eight key components to search for when doing a CBD quality check.

TIP

If you have to work to find important information on the label, the company may well be secretive about other things, too.

Test results (COA)

The *certificate of authenticity*, or COA, is a piece of paperwork that is required in the manufacturing process of any consumer packaged good. Manufacturers must obtain a COA before they can take on an ingredient, thus declaring its origin, safety, and authenticity. Think of literally any ingredient that you may purchase in a grocery store or bodega or online. All the ingredients have associated COAs before they hit the manufacturer's floor. The COA should be by a validated, third-party testing agency, not by the manufacturer of the product.

Providing COAs to consumers is technically required only in the medical and adult-use cannabis spaces. But in the spirit of full disclosure and openness, it has become an industry standard in the CBD space on a national level because brands are looking to build trust with their consumers. For that reason, any brand of note will provide you with a readily accessible COA. For example, it may be in the form of a scannable QR code on a bottle or secondary package, or the retailer may simply hang on to the details of the COA for each batch of the product and make them accessible upon request.

WARNING

If you ever encounter a product without a COA, run. Run like the wind! A COA is the single most identifiable way to determine whether you should continue looking at the product for other degrees of consideration, and a lack of one is a deal-breaker.

Concentration

The concentration is particularly important here because when you're buying CBD to treat a particular condition, you want to make sure you're getting an appropriate product for your needs. A higher concentration CBD product isn't necessarily the best CBD product. On the other hand, a product with a concentration that's too small may not be able to address your condition.

WARNING

If you find a product with a really low price and a very high concentration of CBD, please be skeptical. Concentration and price go hand in hand. Just like you probably wouldn't expect authentic designer quality from a handbag you bought from a hawker on the street, you want to question the quality of the other ingredients in a suspiciously cheap CBD product and whether the claims it's making about the volume of CBD are actually true.

Extraction method

In CBD products, safety is paramount, so transparency on the label about the extraction method is imperative. Look for details about how the CBD was extracted. Different extraction methods mean different things to each consumer. An extraction method like butane or propane results in a higher-volume yield and therefore a lower price point. But the negative trade-off is that extraction methods like these have more unwanted consequences than a more expensive form like double CO_2 processing. A company should be proud to show on its label that it's making the right choice for your health. Chapter 4 has more information about extraction.

Hemp or cannabis

Whether the origin of your CBD product is hemp or cannabis is largely only relevant if you live in a state that disallows cannabis (see the earlier section "Being aware of the laws in your state"). Certain conditions and ailments, such as some neurological conditions, are better treated with a higher concentration of THC than is nationally legal for hemp cannabis. Such treatments are available only from cannabis dispensaries in regulated states.

WARNING

If you have a known adverse reaction to THC, making sure your CBD is hemp-derived and has its THC content accurately labeled is important regardless of what kind of state you live in.

Ingredients

The ingredients used as carriers, bases, or additives in your CBD are as important as the CBD itself. For example, some bases affect CBD's *bioavailability* (your body's ability to receive the CBD more readily). Some ingredients counteract the desired effects of CBD. You wouldn't take a dose of CBD in your caffeinated coffee if your goal was to sleep; similarly, if you're taking CBD as a gut supplement, you probably don't want to consume it in a cookie made with lots of animal fats (butter) and refined sugars.

On the other hand, many complementary ingredients can compound the effects of CBD positively, depending on what you're trying to achieve. Many labels have a section highlighting complementary ingredients front and center to help indicate how effective a product may be at supporting a particular condition. For instance, lavender as an additive to a CBD sleep aid should be incredibly calming and balancing. On the other hand, if you're looking for a pick-me-up, energy-boosting products containing caffeinated substances in addition to the CBD offer you all the benefits of caffeine along with your hemp extract. One of the most popular combinations to date is the addition of turmeric to a CBD tincture for anti-inflammatory properties and pain relief.

Sustainability

Hemp-derived CBD is an agricultural commodity. As the demand increases, so will the technology and capabilities for driving the cost of production down and the profits up. That usually means a decrease in quality, an increase in pesticides, and an inevitable breeding structure for the plant that serves volume over quality.

Anything consumers can do now to support best practices in sustainability in the CBD industry will serve them in the long run. To those ends, here are a few considerations:

>> **Know the origin of your key ingredient, and make sure it's from a reputable source that takes care of the soil, the planet, and, in turn, your body.** Hemp is historically recognized as a *bioremediator,* which means it helps detoxify soils. That's great for the soil, but those toxins go somewhere. Then you have to think about pesticides. Adult-use and medical dispensaries have stringent regulations on organics, but the national market doesn't require organics. (See "Understanding the different kinds of retailers" for more on these sellers.) Most states have regulations that stipulate that minimal amounts of pesticides are acceptable in cannabis. If that's not scary enough, the unscrupulous have used incredible scientific tools and ways to remediate pesticide presence to pass cannabis through the requirements and get it stocked in stores. If you're using a substance for health, you want to take in as few extra toxins as possible in the process.

>> **Understand how packaging can affect the product.** Many of these products are contained in alcohols or oils that interact with the petroleum-based products in their primary packaging. The CBD products you order at home are then shipped across the country to your doorstep. They're inevitably exposed to the elements, creating a higher degree of vulnerability and volatility.

TIP

Stick with glass and recyclable metal packaging wherever possible. When storing something that contains silicone or plastic in the top, avoid laying the product on its side so that the contents don't come into contact with the petroleum-based parts, which degrade over time and will contaminate your product.

Health claims

As I write this, the CBD space itself has an incredible lack of regulation. On a national level, however, FDA guidelines prohibit products in the natural category with no clinical trials or proven medical effectiveness (such as CBD) from claiming to treat any condition or implying it can through imagery and coercive wording.

WARNING

You'll definitely see products as you're browsing the shelves whose manufacturers don't follow these guidelines. Their products don't have some leg up on others; they're likely just not large enough to be caught in the FDA's roundups. And if the FDA isn't catching these companies' illegal claims, consider what other concerning ways they may be flying under the radar.

You'll see statements to the effect of "this product has been shown to help with sleepless nights" or "may be effective against minor inflammation." Other ways around the guidelines include simply naming a product something really literal, like Sleep or Pain, that telegraphs the condition it's supposed to treat. But whether these on-the-nose naming procedures will fly on a larger level is still questionable.

Growing method and location

China is one of the largest producers of hemp, and that very well may mean that it's the largest producer of CBD. That's not as scary as it may initially seem because neither the United States nor China has much if any regulation in the CBD space. But from a sustainability standpoint, is having CBD shipped overseas the most efficient option? (While I'm talking about sustainability, check out the earlier section called — what else? — "Sustainability" for some other important considerations.)

Regardless of the country producing the CBD, the growing method is pretty important, particularly if you're looking for cannabis-derived CBD. You can grow cannabis indoors or outdoors. Modern self-proclaimed connoisseurs tend to prefer indoor varieties because the growers can have more control over the different aspects of the plant that create CBD's specific characteristics and benefits. Environmentalists and some cannabis advocates (and the original growers of the space) argue that, with the right considerations, you can grow great quality product outdoors — with a much more sustainable footprint.

Indoor growing often mimics outdoor variables. For example, growers bring in fans to simulate wind pushing air from side to side. Some indoor growers even include natural sound machines with crickets and birds chirping, all with the idea that outdoor environments serve the quality of growth in a plant.

Outdoor growing, or cultivating rather, allows for a natural relationship to sun and soil as well as all the other animals and elements of nature. Large-scale growing can be more difficult outdoors because the grower has no way to control these elements. Traditionalists, plant medicine workers, herbalists, and many independent growers will tell you that the natural relationship to the environment, as well as the cultivator, is paramount in maintaining the integrity and spirit of the plant. They will also tell you that if you learn how to work with the land, it is easier than synthesizing that relationship at scale in an indoor environment.

Personally, I'm an outdoor kind of gal. I fully support an environment connected to the soil and the sun. Under those circumstances, I trust the process of nature to do its job. (Ideally, it would be in my backyard, but I realize that's not always possible.) Locally grown cannabis is great because it supports a *biome* (biological community) that supports my body, and anything that makes me feel better is a top priority.

Dosing and adjusting appropriately for your needs

When you start using CBD for your particular needs, finding the right dose is important. *Titration* is the process of determining the volume necessary for the intended impact. Really, diving into a bigger dose than necessary just ends up creating larger expense.

REMEMBER

Across cannabis and hemp, ten milligrams is generally considered a baseline dose. Some theories attempt to correlate milligram dosage to body weight, but nothing has been formally agreed upon. Many brands, companies, and advisers alike continue to hang on to the ten-milligram standard, and that's what I use here as an example.

REMEMBER

Most research indicates little possibility of overdosing on CBD. That said, the same research also indicates that most conditions don't require doses over 300 milligrams even for the most severe cases. It's been indicated that humans can't build up a tolerance to CBD, so you don't need to continue increasing your dosage to have the same desired effects; however, after certain high dose usage for extended periods, taking a break is probably best.

MICRODOSING

Microdosing has certainly gotten a lot of attention across the plant medicine space, primarily with cannabis and other psychotropics such as magic mushrooms, or other plants for mental health considerations.

The concept behind *microdosing* is consistently adding a concentration of a substance to your bloodstream so that you have consistent and mild levels of the intended effect rather than taking larger doses and having concentrated effects all at once for a shorter time.

If your CBD products come from a medical or adult-use dispensary and have a concentration of THC, microdosing may be a conversation for you. Presumably, the CBD-only version of microdosing would align with supplementations, and the benefits would be like those of taking a vitamin to help maintain a level quality of health.

Think of ten milligrams as a supplemental dosage — something you take to just maintain a level of health and quality of life. Try that dosage for three days; if you don't feel, see, or have any indication that it's having the effects you want it to (beyond supplementation), you may want to slowly dose up. By that, I mean incrementally adding five milligrams at a time until you do see the effects.

REMEMBER

At each level of dosing, give your body at least three days to adjust to determine whether that dose is accurate. I can understand being eager to get the effects you're after, but when introducing something new to your body, you need to give it time to react and enter your bloodstream for maximum effect.

Tapping into Online Distributors

Reputability is far more complex in the digital landscape simply because you get no human-to-human interaction. It feels like online sources have less accountability, and they're just as likely to be misleading or fraudulent as brick-and-mortar companies are. Of course, you can find plenty of highly reputable sources in the online sphere. (In fact, I own one of those sources.)

REMEMBER

Ask the same questions you would when reading labels in person (see the earlier section "Checking quality"). You should absolutely be able to easily access the certificates of authenticity and the test results for the quality and concentration of the CBD in your product with a simple click of a button or a quick request to the supplier of the site.

TIP

When buying online, consider buying from the country you're based in to make purchasing and receiving a product easier and to give you more recourse if something goes wrong with your order. (Outside your own jurisdiction, you typically have fewer options for setting a bad situation right.) So if you're based in the United States, think about buying from a U.S source.

Choosing an online seller

By reading even a little bit of this book, you probably know more about CBD than even some of the retailers selling the product. CBD is such a hot-ticket item that people realize the value of moving quickly to sell products and don't always take the time to invest in learning about each individual product, how to sell it, what it's good for, and who it's good for.

The best online CBD sources are going to be the most transparent sources giving you clear COAs and proof points about the brands and companies that they're selling and supporting. (Head to the earlier section "Test results (COA)" for details on this document.) As a proprietor and creator, I've seen a lot of companies come and go. I truly believe the ones that have longevity are the ones that take customer care seriously and that are available for you with a phone call. Personally, I like to see stories and content around the brands. I also value founder stories that support why and how somebody created the company along with its investments and community — sustainability as a strong business that supports its customers. If a retailer can share that information with you in a clear way that makes you feel like its product is also going to address the ailments you're specifically shopping to treat, you're probably barking up the right tree.

Also consider whether a retailer seems like the community for you — that is, do the people feel like they're your people? You see so many different kinds of styles across internet retailers, with vibes ranging from premier and prestige to mainstream and accessible to hip and millennial. The people who created the site you're shopping on have likely crafted a brand personality that reveals which vibe they fall under. Think of their website as an aesthetic introduction to their marketplace.

Here are some of my favorite online sources:

>> `Shop-poplar.com`: My own online platform, Poplar, which focuses on all-natural remedies for pain, stress, and sleep, carries a wide variety of CBD brands I believe represent the deepest integrity in the space. We also carry diverse plant and mineral medicine without CBD because CBD isn't a one-size-fits- all product.

>> `Humblebloom.com`: A marketplace driven by equity in cannabis, selling exclusively CBD products, does a nice job of honoring community and addressing historical, cultural, and political injustices in cannabis.

>> `Fleurmarche.com`: A site driven by the female purchasing audience and selling CBD products exclusively curates premium brands and sells their own products.

>> `Missgrass.com`: One of the earliest cannabis-focused female lenses on the scene. It has recently released CBD products exclusively while working to build out its THC product line for California and a whole host of others designed specifically for a broader audience in the middle market with names too numerous to mention.

REMEMBER

There are, of course, exceptions. If you encounter outlets that are a little bit more salesy and offer you regular subscription service with incredibly deep discounts for buying larger volume over a committed period, they may have an agenda. They're likely hoping to get you committed to something that you'll forget to cancel or that isn't very effective. If their product model is to keep you trapped in the cycle by continued payment processing, what does that tell you? That the product isn't compelling enough to keep you wanting to come back for more.

Tracing the path of the best sellers

Right now, the best sellers in the online space are the ones that can get to the top of the marketing food chain the fastest — who understands the marketing funnels and who has the largest marketing budget. So who's the best? I think the cream will rise to the top. Eventually. For now, I would tend to believe the resources that you've been using for your groceries, your skin care, and other products. If these sites you trust have started to bring in products containing CBD, they likely carry CBD products with the same level of consideration and trust factors that are important to you.

The other piece of this issue is that some retailers almost exclusively sell CBD products or products specifically designed around the health and wellness space. As long as these companies have an expert at their fingertips to help them develop their product portfolios and to help the consumer understand how to best serve themselves with these products, they should be quality resources.

BUYING RETAIL PRODUCTS ENHANCED WITH CBD

As the market continues to evolve, many random products are going to just add CBD for the heck of it. Inevitably, CBD will be just another ingredient alongside goji berries, oats, and bee pollen. As I write this, the marketplace seems to be dominated by companies selling CBD products with other ingredients, but I think a flip is coming where products will be sold with CBD as an ingredient and not the driving force on the label.

Remember: CBD has a lot of beneficial functions in the body, as I discuss in Chapter 3. But in some products, the only real purpose it serves is as a marketing ploy. Use your personal judgment to decide, say, whether a CBD-infused pillowcase can improve your sleep.

Being an Informed Consumer

In the end, making a decision that best serves you is up to you. This is your body and your health, and being as informed as possible is the best way to make a good decision.

This book represents what I've learned in my 17 years of experience in the cannabis industry. But the information about this industry evolves daily, so by the time this book is published the industry may likely have had the opportunity to explore a bit more deeply into your particular condition or ailment. It's your job to stay informed.

Being wary of CBD scams

The CBD industry seems ripe for scammers. The most common scam is claiming there is CBD, especially a high volume, in a product, but in reality that product has less CBD than it claims or none at all. Sadly, as a consumer, you won't know, as there are few checks and balances. That is why I like the process of buying through a marketplace that specializes in medicine, or CBD medicine specifically, because the marketplace serves as another checks-and-balance system to validate the claims of ingredients and concentration in the products.

One of the safest bets to check not only the products but also the retailers is to determine whether your product has been third-party tested and validated with a legitimate COA. That data should be readily available to you upon request. If it's not, say goodbye to that particular product. Also worth noting is whether the testing agency listed on the third-party test and paperwork is a validated party, which should be a pretty quick online search, confirming the validity of the testing agency. Again, this is something the retailer should have already done for you.

Keep your eyes open. Read your labels. Trust your gut.

Avoiding pitfalls

Your local gas station or corner store may not be the best place to buy something you're using to treat a medical condition. Consider largely the kind of proprietor or store that you'd trust, and only buy from such establishments.

If you can buy from somebody you know, chances are you're going to avoid the pitfalls and potential hazards of buying snake oil. So ask around! Undoubtedly, you have a friend or two who already uses CBD oil for one thing or another and who may be able to give you recommendations or referrals for reputable sellers. I promise you that you have nothing to be ashamed of in talking about cannabis.

Chapter 7

Delving into Forms and Delivery Systems

As I explain in Chapter 4, you can choose from so many different kinds of CBD extracts, ranging from full-spectrum down to the isolated molecule. Reviewing your options before choosing your ideal type of extract and delivery method is important because each of these CBD extracts can be used in different forms.

This chapter explores the forms of CBD extracts and why each of them is uniquely valuable. I also discuss different ways you can consume these extracts.

Becoming Familiar with the Forms of CBD

The forms of CBD extracts range from a full-spectrum, which contains almost all the plant matter and chemicals, to an isolate that contains only the isolated molecule of CBD. Each form of extract has different implications.

The form that makes you feel most comfortable and gives you what you need is inevitably the right form for you.

As I discuss in Chapter 2, many people subscribe to the *entourage effect* — the idea that the different *cannabinoids* and *terpenes* (plant chemicals) in cannabis interact with one another and work best as a team. In treating some conditions, these interactions do lead to a better result, and remedies that stick closely to the whole-plant form are preferable. You can get the intended effects for some conditions from CBD on its own, and for still others, combining CBD with other ingredients (guest stars, if you will) in a product maximizes potency.

Different theories exist in the scientific community that suggest the importance of these different extracts and methods. But as of this writing, that's all they are: plain old theories.

The following sections provide you with the basics on each of the six most common forms of CBD.

Full-spectrum

Full-spectrum CBD extract contains everything from the plant but the fiber. For CBD, full-spectrum extract usually comes from the hemp plant rather than the cannabis plant because of the legal limits (0.3 percent) on THC in CBD. Getting a full-spectrum extract that meets this standard from a THC-containing cannabis plant would be difficult.

That said, full-spectrum extracts exist across the entire cannabis spectrum. Regulated dispensaries (see Chapter 6), from adult-use to medical, have a wide range of full-spectrum extracts with varying concentrations of CBD, THC, and other cannabinoids.

Full-spectrum has gained a lot of attention specifically because predominant theories in the cannabis space suggest that CBD's benefits are magnified, or their reach potentially broadened, because of all the minor cannabinoids, flavonoids, and terpenes present in a full spectrum extract. Check out www.cannabistech. com/articles/what-is-the-entourage-effect-in-cannabis/ to find out more.

Broad-spectrum

Broad-spectrum CBD extract contains almost all the plant chemicals and constituents. But it's missing one key factor. The reason broad-spectrum is so common is the desire to keep the plant as close to full as possible in the extract form thanks to the legal issues with THC. The result is a broad-spectrum product that contains all the chemicals except THC.

TECHNICAL STUFF

It's actually a little bit more complicated than that; realistically, it's an extract that removes the plant chemicals from the fiber and then in a secondary step removes the THC down to a 0.3 percent concentration, leaving only their remaining plant chemicals with high concentrations of CBD.

Distillate

One step farther down the line from broad-spectrum (see the preceding section) is *distillate*. It's a further distilled version of broad-spectrum where more of the plant chemicals are removed so that the focus is on CBD (or, in other applications, any specific cannabinoid). A defining feature of distillate is a high concentration of cannabinoids. Because of market demand and increased interest, it's quite popular.

Note: The removal of various other chemicals from distillate affects its color. It often appears amber to light yellow and can be denser than the two forms in the preceding sections.

Isolate

Isolate is exactly that: the isolated chemical compound of CBD. Distilling the cannabis extract over and over again (in a process a bit more complicated than that) leaves an isolated molecule. That molecule appears to be in a yellow-tinted (sometimes white) crystalline form. You may find it ground to look like a fine powder when it's sold on its own in the open market.

REMEMBER

Distilling a chemical down to 100 percent purity is nearly impossible. So lab results and test results show 99.9 percent CBD isolate with remaining compounds either from the extraction process or from the plant itself. This remaining 0.1 percent can include terpenes, flavonoids, or other cannabinoids.

Isolate in and of itself doesn't have any of the perceived benefits of the entourage effect. However, formulators and those interested in the future evolution of CBD prize it because it's so easy to apply into a formula and straightforwardly determine the resulting effectiveness.

Wax, rosin, and so on

This style of extract is one of the purest forms of extract. The nicknames seem endless: wax, rosin, shatter, sap, and glass (just to name a few). So do the options for consumption.

Waxes and rosins are useable individually and as additives. As additives, the end goal is to increase the potency of a product. After all, waxes and rosins are prized specifically for being the most potent and most consistent of all the extracts.

The names are often representative of the form and appearance. Glass, for example, is clear and has more of a crystalline, glasslike structure. It's less opaque than wax but still has less color than other variations of extracts. Various other forms come in colors from light yellow to burned amber.

Hash and kief

The most original of the extracts may be hash and kief. They have long histories across cultures as being the additives of choice beyond just flower in and of itself. *Kief* is the *trichomes* (small, hairlike growths) that have been separated from the plant matter. These are also known as the resin glands of the cannabis flower.

Kief is technically the stage before hash. As kief undergoes pasteurization through heating, it turns into *hash.* Hash itself has no one true shape. It can be a slightly pliable ball, brick, coin, or numerous other shapes made for stylistic purposes and accessibility. Like wax or rosin (see the preceding section), it's often an additive in separate products to add value. But it can be used on its own.

Uncovering the Delivery Systems

You can encounter so many drastically different delivery systems for cannabis and CBD. Which system you choose is important because using this chemical as a medicine requires you to seriously consider the condition you're treating and how the delivery system affects that ailment specifically. As a natural medicine, CBD has variables that affect each individual's body differently, and delivery system can play into that as well.

Each method has a different onset time (see Table 7-1), uptake qualities, and implications for how long the effects last. For instance, if you want quicker relief, you may be inclined to smoke or inhale CBD because this approach has a faster uptake.

TABLE 7-1   **Onset Times for Different Forms of CBD Delivery**

Form	Onset Times
Smoking and inhalation	A few minutes.
Sublinguals	Immediate to 30 minutes.
Edibles and capsules	Between 30 minutes and 2 hours. This time range depends on how full your stomach already is because the CBD enters through your digestive tract.
Transdermal patches	Anywhere from 15 to 30 minutes.
Topicals	Between 30 and 45 minutes. Remember that some formulations have immediate sensory effects because of a combination of other powerful ingredients.

TIP

If you're looking for an immediate onset but also need a longer duration, you may need a multifaceted solution, such as layering something inhalable and something edible. Edibles tend to have longer onset times and less bioavailability, so something stronger may be necessary. However, they last for longer periods. Examples of these situations include someone who needs help both falling asleep and then staying asleep and someone with acute pain who needs both immediate and ongoing relief.

In this section, I introduce you to the various delivery forms available. The remaining sections in the chapter cover each delivery form in more detail.

Smoking

One of the oldest and probably most loved forms of consumption is smoking. Across the space, smoking is still the most common way to consume cannabis as a whole, perhaps in part because it has the allure and the tradition of cannabis and marijuana culture. CBD, specifically, lives in a slightly different category of rate of consumption because of the number of topicals on the marketplace; you can read about topicals later in the chapter. With smoking, the bioavailability is high and the onset times are almost immediate, so when you reach for something smokable, you know what you're getting.

Vaping

Vaping has a lot of the same properties as smoking. However, it has the benefit of a very high heat vaporizing a flower or a distillate, resulting in an immediate-onset, smoke-free experience. Vaping has gotten a bad reputation; when you're vaping a distillate, the product often has a filler or base oil. Many of the companies diving into this market did little research on the effects of these base oils or added flavors, and the backlash has been enormous.

Dabbing

Dabbing is essentially a super-high-heat form of inhaling wax, resin, or the like. The vapors provide a quick onset and intense cannabinoid experience. The effects are short-lived but much deeper than many other forms of consumption.

Dabbing appeals to those who consider themselves deep into the space of cannabis and to a specific subset of the community that requires really high concentrations of cannabinoids, specifically for the treatment of difficult to address conditions such as cancer.

Sublinguals

Sublinguals are second in popularity only to smoking and vaping. *Sublinguals* directly interact with the blood vessels under your tongue. With sublinguals, the idea is to place the concentrated extracts under your tongue and hold them in place until the blood vessels in your mouth are able to absorb them. Consequently, the interaction creates a more immediate onset than other forms of consumption.

Sublinguals have two common variations:

>> An extract done in alcohol, is technically called a *tincture*.

>> An oil-based extract is referred to as oil-based sublingual or a sublingual.

Additional, less popular forms available are nanoparticulated CBD tinctures, which could be either alcohol, oil, or water-based tinctures. The term *nanoparticulated* suggests that the CBD itself has been made nano — or smaller — making it more easily absorbed into the body. Some tinctures say water-soluble on the packaging, implying that it is even more easily absorbed into the body (the justification being that because our bodies are mainly water, like with like is more effective).

Eating and drinking

Eating and drinking CBD products basically have the same properties, though the methods are slightly different. Consumption of food-based products requires that your body metabolize the CBD through your stomach lining. In other words, it gets absorbed from the lining of your stomach and into the bloodstream like other nutrients do. Of course, the foods in question can be anything, including hemp byproducts like seeds, hemp hearts, or extracted hemp protein.

REMEMBER

All the goods have to pass through your stomach acid and into your stomach, which can compromise their bioavailability. It can also affect uptake time, so be sure to set aside a generous amount of time for edibles. Ask yourself, "Do I have a 30-minute-to-two-hour window?" Beverages can take a little less time because they have less fiber and particles for your body to process before it can absorb all the nutrients.

Topicals

Topicals are designed to address localized considerations like skin stress or acute pain. Some topicals are also designed for sleep assistance. They're in a league of their own because they play with a completely different receptor base. (Unless you're talking about transdermal patches or transdermal topicals, which I discuss in the later section "Touching on Topical and Transdermal Applications.")

Most topicals are, well, just topical. They don't reach into the bloodstream because penetration through the skin is a complicated process. The formulations in most CBD products are in their infancy, so not many on the marketplace can address or penetrate on a deeper level.

Topical products come in different varieties. For example, some exist in oils; others are lotion or cream-based, and still others are balms and salves.

Choosing Your Smoking or Inhalation Method

Smoking is primarily the most efficient way to feel the effects of CBD as quickly as possible. Some people find some aspects or consequences of the process less than desirable, but for others, those are the pieces that make it interesting. Smoking flower, for instance, has all of the pieces of packing the bowl or rolling the joint, and it's very hands-on. You may find that selecting your particular flower based on scent, feel, and origin is deeply intimate. It depends on your own connection to nature and feelings about sensory experiences. But if you're trying to make the process simple, those extra steps may feel overwhelming. Other variations of smoking, such as vaping and dabbing, can eliminate some of those aspects and variables that come with straightforward smoking.

Up to half of the cannabinoid content that you're consuming via smoking and inhalation is going to be accessible to your bloodstream. Therefore, you may need less CBD than if you were using a transdermal patch or an edible.

REMEMBER

Smoking CBD is a bit like applying red lipstick before you eat. The effect is great and nearly immediate, but the ideal result is brief. You can expect the effects of smoking CBD to last for up to three hours.

Smoking, vaping, or dabbing?

The variables that are a part of your selection process in smoking, vaping, or dabbing include the following:

>> **The type of flower or extracts:** Or, in the case of dabbing, the formation.

>> **The type of device.**

>> **The location, setting, and dosage:** You can make assumptions about the dose and concentration of what you're consuming when you smoke flower. After all, half a joint is a visually measurable amount. But vaping and dabbing allow for a bit more of a metered experience.

Deciding on a device for smoking flower

Flower is the ultimate way to experience full-spectrum plant effects. Flower offers opportunities that extracts and modified versions of the flower may not. The plant itself contains hundreds of beneficial plant chemicals.

TIP

Smell it. Does it resonate with you? Terpenes that are responsible for much of the flower's scent also have incredible therapeutic properties. They're what the essential oil aromatherapy industry relies on heavily. So the scent of the terpenes will "speak" to you. Trust them.

SET AND SETTING

Set and setting are important pieces of the experiential puzzle, so you should consider your physical and social environments. These aspects of consumption can round out, amplify, or moderate your experience. The conversation around set and setting largely evolved out of the psychedelic experience. But because cannabis is a psychedelic-containing plant when THC comes into play, it's an important conversation to have.

Your device of choice matters when you're smoking flower.

- **Paper:** The combustion of paper creates some side effects, such as a harsh feeling on the lungs or in the throat. If you're going to smoke paper, natural products like rice papers may be a better try.

- **Pipe:** Pipes are a little bit more direct. They exist in colorful glass or crystal iterations called *bubblers,* and then of course you have *bongs,* all of which run the smoke through water. This process almost acts as a filtration process, clarifying it for the lungs.

- **Vaporizer:** Vaporizers use a higher heat method. Combustion produces vapor rather than standard smoke. Allegedly, the vapor is the easiest on the lungs.

Picking a pre-roll

Pre-rolls are rolled-up flower and various other things. Picking a pre-roll can be much like picking a flower plus any flavor customizations.

TIP

If you prefer something that's rolled by somebody else, make sure it's rolled with full flower. Sure, not having to roll your own joints or flower is great, but the caveat is that you can't see what's in the roll as easily. What often gets rolled up in these bad boys can be harsher on your lungs and contain less of the good stuff. Plus, they often have added synthetic flavors. (Do you really want the experience of blueberries or a melted taffy on top of your cannabis-scented cigarette?) Waxes, kief, hash, and so forth have the specific purposes of increasing the concentrations of pre-rolls. Sticking with full flower helps keep you from consuming subpar products.

Because flower, smoking, and joints aren't really going anywhere in the full-spectrum and CBD spaces, lots of incredible brands are coming to the table with pre-roll options made from full flower. So they're out there; you just have to make sure to do the proper digging.

Deciding to vape

If you're going to smoke and you're not attached to the flower part of the experience, vaping is a great alternative. I'd say it's the preferable alternative if you need a quick and easy onset. This method produces no smoke because of the type of high-heat combustion. You're not affecting those around you as much, so vaping is great for discretion, ease, and function.

TIP

You can choose from a variety of devices for vaping:

>> If you want to vape flower, get an in-home device that's top of the line; you'll be happy you did.

>> If you're looking for a pen and relevant accessories, you have a lot of cartridge options. For longevity, buy a good-quality pen. Here are a couple of other considerations:

- Choose a cartridge that comes from a natural, organic provider that preferably doesn't use any carrier oils. That may mean that your cartridge has a little less viscosity, which translates to a more challenging pull from your pen.

- Your cartridge may also require a consistently higher heat level. Also, do a quick Google search on how to use a lighter to heat the vape cartridge for ease of function.

Dabbing CBD

Dabbing is largely a social form of consumption. And by social, I mean young, cool, hip, intense . . . you catch my drift.

REMEMBER

CBD is a remedy more than a recreational cannabinoid. Some need it in very high concentrations to address the severity of their symptoms and challenging conditions.

VAPEGATE

Vapegate was the overarching media frenzy in 2019 around the effects of flavored tobacco vaporizing devices with young adults and teens as well as vaping's meteoric rise to popularity. Vape-related illnesses and some deaths were sweeping through this consumption community, which understandably had a rippling effect through the cannabis community. Consequently, new regulations and limited insurance available for brands selling CBD vape products have been the aftereffect.

Still, vaping is here to stay. Now some standards exist for the materials you're using to vape so that you're not inhaling harmful adhesives, plastics, and the like. Ask yourself whether the additives going into these products (like the base oils) are safe for combustion. And if so, what happens in your lungs when you consume perpetual doses of such materials? The point is that Vapegate allowed vapers to choose more wisely and simultaneously challenged companies to do better by them.

Concentrated pain experiences, high anxiety that can lead to panic attacks, and consistent or severe sleeplessness may all be perfect reasons to consider dabbing CBD. As with any form of extract, the strain and variety of cannabis are an important consideration. (Flip to Chapter 2 for the lowdown on strains and varieties.) Make sure to check the terpenes, the cannabinoid content, and the COAs (certificates of authenticity; see Chapter 6) to make sure that what you're dabbing is appropriate for whatever condition you're addressing.

Touching on Topical and Transdermal Applications

Topicals are a really interesting conversation point. Their uniqueness stems from the fact that they don't fall neatly into the categorical conversation of interaction with the endocannabinoid system. As Chapter 3 explains, the system that's internal to our bodies, the endocannabinoid system (ECS), is reminiscent of the cannabinoid system of the cannabis plant. Topicals have the incredible capability of interacting with a variety of other systems and the receptors in our skin. Your skin has a notable number of receptors that interact with CBD!

Smoothing on skin

A variety of forms within the topicals category can be applied directly to the skin: creams, lotions, salves, balms, oils, and serums. The major differences among these forms are in the other components of the products.

>> **Balms and salves:** These products (which are less viscous) have textures ranging from honey to hockey pucks. They're strictly oil-based formulas. They have the bonus of being easier to produce because CBD is a lipid, which means it's oil soluble. They are largely for first aid, from pain to cuts and wound care. They can also be deeply nourishing skin and body care products, but because of their density they tend to require a bit of working into the skin for penetration.

>> **Lotions and creams:** These options are largely water-based. Their formulas require some sort or emulsifier or *solubilizer* (something to make it more dissolvable) to incorporate the CBD. Formulations that have a water base are more susceptible to contamination from outside elements that can compromise the quality and the effectiveness of the products. These products are softer and lighter to the touch. As a result, they appear more in the skincare space than the pain relief space because they address skin stressors rather than pain.

>> **Oils and serums:** These products are more like vitamins and nutrients designed to be delivered into the skin in an oil lipid-based formula. They often have to gradually soak into the skin. They can be a little bit less complicated to manufacture, in part because they're less likely to become contaminated. In this way, they differ from products with water bases. You typically see them in the skincare market focusing on body care and massages.

Because balms and salves are thicker, they require more of a massage technique to apply than lotions and creams do. That technique alone improves *microcirculation* (circulation in the smallest blood vessels), which helps reduce inflammation and compounds or assists the intended benefits of CBD such as antimicrobial, antibacterial, and antifungal properties. Regardless of the application process, oils and serums fall somewhere between the salves/balms and the lotions/creams and require a little bit more work from a penetration perspective.

The facial oils and the serums (because of their manufacturing ease) are some of the first to hit the market with CBD skincare, so you'll probably see more of them from a great diversity of brands.

REMEMBER

High supply doesn't correlate with superb quality. With facial skincare in particular, you want to be really aware of the additional ingredients and whether these compounds in their concentrations are active or just for fluff.

Pasting on patches

Direct access to the bloodstream will always be the best way to introduce medicine with fewer side effects and increased bioavailability. That's where patches come in.

In order for a patch to be effective, it must be designed with transdermal properties. As I discuss in Chapter 1, *transdermal* means that the formulation reaches into the bloodstream. The skin is a complex structure designed to protect the body and your delicate insides. It's a giant barrier meant to keep things out, so products that want to penetrate into the bloodstream and circulate throughout the body have to have some sort of penetrating agents to gain access.

They do so by creating microcuts or abrasions in the skin. Think about when you brush up against a stinging nettle plant and it creates an itching, burning sensation. That sensation occurs because the plant surface has made microcuts in your skin and then the plant oils have penetrated, creating a reaction. Transdermal patches for pain relief are popular in traditional Chinese medicine.

As with any CBD product, you need to pay incredible attention to the number of active ingredients in a transdermal patch to know whether it'll work. The penetrating agents in transdermals are often petroleum-based. When you're looking for effectiveness and some sort of relief, that may not be a big concern. I personally tend to steer clear.

I believe we're going to see this category of transdermal patches grow tremendously as the science around advocacy in CBD evolves.

Spraying on CBD

Across the market, you're going to see various kinds of sprayable CBD, from oils to hydrosols. *Hydrosols* are water-based. They may be *nanoparticulated* (which means the molecules are suspended in a water base) or a combination of water and oils with a suspension agent.

From a skincare perspective, the *hydrogels* (water-based gels) and hydrosols make a lot of sense. They're handy because of their ability to layer with other skincare products; you can easily integrate them into your daily routine.

Products in the pain category aren't nearly as common, but they're proving to be incredibly desirable. Apothecanna, a leading topical brand in the United States, found that customers were drawn largely to its fast-drying formulas. Its products are easily sprayable. Not only did the spray nozzle allow for users to hit hard-to-reach areas like the neck and lower back, but the fast-absorbing action also made for a quick result.

Taking CBD Orally

From chewing gummies to drinking CBD beverages, you have so many ways to incorporate CBD into your routine orally. This category is undoubtedly the most popular one for product manufacturers (because of the diverse, widespread opportunities to create fun, interesting products), so choosing isn't always easy.

The following sections break down some popular methods for taking CBD orally.

Putting CBD under your tongue

Taking CBD *sublingually* (under your tongue) is second to smoking and vaping CBD in terms of rapid onset time. (You can read about smoking and vaping earlier in the chapter.) That's because the blood vessels under your tongue allow for more immediate uptake into the bloodstream. The idea is to let the product sit under your tongue for 30 to 90 seconds, if you can, for maximum intake. You can expect results (if you're actually going for a sensation) in as little as 10 minutes and up to 30 minutes.

WHAT IS BIOAVAILABILITY?

One of the important things to note when using CBD, or any medicine for that matter, is the bioavailability. *Bioavailability* refers to the amount of a substance that gets into the circulating blood of the body. The reason bioavailability is important because the amount of the substance will determine the active effects on the body. The bioavailability of a substance is different for every form factor, from inhalation to sublingual and edible to topical. The following chart illustrates the bioavailability of CBD in the various form factors that are available on the market. It shares just how much CBD you can expect to experience.

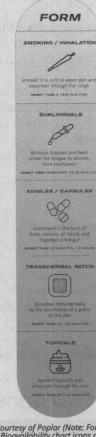

Courtesy of Poplar (Note: Form Bioavailability chart icons are made by Those Icons, turkkup, DinosoftLabs, and Freepik, from www.flaticon.com.*)*

Despite its quicker onset, sublingual CBD doesn't necessarily last as long as other forms. The results can last up to three hours (or more), depending on the doses and the severity of whatever condition that you're trying to treat.

You can find sublinguals with a variety of bases:

>> **Oil:** Oil bases are quite popular because the lipid form of the CBD molecule makes the two easily compatible.

>> **Alcohol:** Alcohol-based sublinguals often have a concentration of glycerin to ease the sublingual feeling in the mouth. These options are historically the most common sublinguals; you may know them as *tinctures*. Because of the alcohol extraction component, the development process for these products has one fewer piece.

>> **Water:** The water-soluble option stems from the philosophy that these products uptake into the body more quickly and easily because the human body is technically 60 percent water with vital organs being closer to 70-80 percent water. This theory is unproven across the CBD space in terms of increased effectiveness, but that doesn't keep companies from continuing to develop in that space.

>> **Nanoparticulated:** The nanoparticulated form suspended in water or oil is also a move to suggest that more CBD becomes accessible to the body because the small particle form is easier for the body to absorb.

Sublinguals also come in various forms of extracts, from broad-spectrum to full-spectrum to isolate. (See Chapter 4 for more on extracts.) These aspects are important considerations because different extracts are good for different things. The same goes for the concentrations of the CBD and the other components in a sublingual, so look carefully at the labels to determine whether the quantities of what you want are present and at what concentration. A good (that is, reputable) production company should have this info readily available.

Because of the popularity of sublinguals and their lack of complexity, the market-place is chock full of sublingual products that contain lots of other components designed to mask flavors or enhance properties. Your personal priorities determine which of these factors is more important to you. If you're looking for the best product for a particular need, you may focus on sublinguals that enhance the CBD benefits you need and not worry so much about the flavors. On the other hand, if you're sensitive specifically to the taste and smell of CBD flower, you may want a little bit of flavoring in there.

Good companies often address flavoring and effectiveness in one swoop. You can find additions that kill two birds with one stone, like peppermint and orange oils. These particular essential oils contain properties that can compound with the terpene profiles of cannabis flower.

Chewing gummies, tapes, mints, and more

If you find sublinguals (see the preceding section) to be a little off-putting, chewable gummies, mints, and the like are a great opportunity to get similar benefits in a different form. Chewing gum, or something similar, for an extended period — to the point where it almost dissolves in your mouth and liquefies — allows access to those same blood vessels under your tongue that sublinguals use. Chewable forms tend to have more familiar, enjoyable (versus medicinal) flavor profiles, so depending on your preferences, they may be easier or more palatable to consume. You can throw a chewable mint in your bag or wallet and easily take it with you on the go. Many of these products also come with complementary ingredient combinations and small doses.

Because the manufacturing for these types of goods is so sophisticated, you see a variation from medical and adult-use dispensaries, especially from state to state. Chapter 6 has more on dispensaries. However, on a national level, you're more likely to see uniformity and a deeper variety of forms with hemp-derived, CBD-focused brands across the spectrum. Gummies tend to be one of the most popular forms, probably because they're so reminiscent of gummy treats for kids. In any case, just a quick internet search turns up tons of brands.

If you don't like high concentrations of sugar, look for products that are free of corn syrup. Instead, check the ingredients list for all-natural sugars. So many complementary ingredients can create really interesting flavor profiles with a touch of sweetness. To be clear, sugar doesn't inhibit or negatively interact with CBD. However, regularly consuming CBD chewables means you'll be munching candies consistently, and that sugar can add up.

Cooking with CBD

Cooking with CBD can be an awesome form of supplementation. Getting a whole hemp profile into the digestive system offers incredible opportunities. You can cook with hemp hearts and hemp seeds. Don't be afraid to use hemp flower, hemp flour, hemp mylk, and any number of other hemp products that allow for a more holistic approach to the nutritional and supplemental aspects of hemp and CBD. Nutritionists and doctors alike have said that CBD's benefits to the endocannabinoid system are most accessible and effective when you include the whole plant protein fiber in your diet.

Many of the hemp supplements you find can be contained in a hemp seed oil, which partly addresses the whole-plant issue but not entirely. More frequently, you find full-spectrum hemp extract added to a base oil. Base oils range from MCT oil (*medium-chain triglyceride* oil, which is a derivative of coconuts and palms) to olive oil and grapeseed oil. You can use all these hemp-added oils as additives for cooking. Some of them are actually specifically designed for enhancing meals.

TIP

Potli CBD-infused olive oil is a great addition because it's quite clear what you're getting, and most people know how to use olive oil. Use it fresh as a topping or in a salad dressing instead of heating it, which can compromise the integrity of the olive oil or the CBD.

REMEMBER

Heating any supplemental CBD in the cooking process can degrade the valuable properties in the plant extract itself. To stay safe, use these products as a finishing touch rather than a cooked ingredient. Another option is to keep your temperatures below 350 degrees Fahrenheit and limit cooking times to less than an hour.

Baking with cannabis is an age-old tradition. You've probably heard stories from your friend's parents about pot cookies "back in the day," but you can get the desired benefits of CBD without the high of pot cookies. You can find recipes galore that include processes on how to create just the form you need for your baking, whether you're starting from flower and creating your own oil or buying something off the shelf.

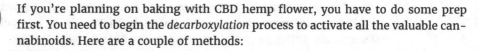

TIP

If you're planning on baking with CBD hemp flower, you have to do some prep first. You need to begin the *decarboxylation* process to activate all the valuable cannabinoids. Here are a couple of methods:

>> To decarboxylate your hemp flower in the oven, spread it out across a cookie sheet. Preheat your oven to 225 degrees Fahrenheit and when it has reached the ideal temperature, put the flower in the oven essentially toasting the cannabis for 45 minutes. The middle rack is best for more even flow and heat. If the flower seems like it may be cooking too quickly or browning, turn down the heat a bit.

>> For a slow cooker, simply add your flower and your oil-based carrier to the cooker, put a lid on it, and cook it on low heat (200 degrees Fahrenheit) for up to three hours, being sure to stir occasionally. Your carrier should turn a vibrant greenish color with maybe a slight touch of yellowish-brown. Definitely don't let it get dark brown; that means it's beyond toasted and approaching burned, which not only compromises vital nutrients but also tastes quite bad. If you don't trust your slow cooker, add a touch of water; it'll evaporate in the process.

Swallowing CBD in pill form

Pills are familiar supplements, and they come in many recognizable versions: packed pills, gel caps filled with powder or liquid, or soft gels that have squishy, gelatinous shells around an oil base. These forms have long been popular across the CBD/cannabis spectrum.

From a CBD supplementation standpoint, pills can be quite simple to incorporate into your daily routine, especially if that routine already includes pills. You can just add another one and know that you're getting what you need.

REMEMBER

Know, though, that pills certainly fall low on the spectrum of bioavailability (because the pill has to penetrate your stomach acid and go through the lining of your stomach), which means you may need higher doses to get you as far as you need to go. You can anticipate at least a 30 percent reduction in overall concentration by the time the CBD hits your bloodstream.

Figuring out exactly what dose is the right dose in a pill form can require a little back and forth maneuvering. Sometimes the tweaking process involves taking a dosage high enough to make you feel like your condition is being alleviated and then dialing it back a little bit to see whether you can use less and have the same intended effects. Taking more than is required is expensive and unnecessary.

Some CBD pills on the market contain value-added ingredients specific to certain conditions. The most common examples are turmeric and capsaicin for both pain relief and inflammation. You may also see melatonin as a popular additive for sleep aids. Different combinations of cannabinoids paired with concentrations of CBD are even starting to roll out. For instance, Cannabinol (CBN) is becoming more visible as a sleep supplement. The preliminary research suggests that this duo may be one of the best ways to address sleep issues.

As with any reputable CBD product, the labels of CBD pill supplements should give you really thorough details about the what, why, and how. Look for something that's clearly presented so you feel like you can trust the company.

Chapter **8**

Using CBD Safely and Responsibly

The commercialization of the CBD industry has a fortunate upside: It has created so much more safety and responsibility for not just those driving the boat but also for the passengers, like you. The opportunity to explore new products and delivery methods is abundant. Of course, the process still does require a degree of consideration on your side. Safely engaging with CBD doesn't just mean knowing the product source and making sure that the supplier is trustworthy. It also means knowing what an optimal dose looks and feels like for you.

This chapter is really a way for you to get the best bang for your buck. I help you explore potency, dosing, and what is right for your body. Additionally, I expand upon how to best consume in a way that serves your lifestyle without compromising others — CBD etiquette, if you will. I also walk you through further exploration of actions, interactions, and efficacy of CBD, so that you can optimize your outcomes as efficiently as possible.

Figuring Out How Much to Take

If you're looking for consumer-facing hard science about what dose is right for what condition, you'll be sorely disappointed. Accessible information just doesn't exist for a lot of this stuff, so the best thing I can tell you is to start slow.

TIP

Starting with a dose that's lower than what you may need poses little risk of potential harm. From there, you can work your way up to the ideal concentration.

This section covers all the details around potency and bioavailability so you can start to understand your dose. It also covers daily dosing and working your chosen form into your schedule.

Adjusting for product potency

Potency is one of the most important considerations and should be labeled front and center on any product that you're consuming.

WARNING

I highly recommend staying away from any CBD product that someone gives you with no written record of its supposed potency.

Most brands highlight their product potency, because doing so is good business if you want to be shelf-worthy in an industry with incredible competition. Carefully look on the front label of any prospective CBD product (see Figure 8-1) for this information. If it's not there, or you have to strain to find it, be wary.

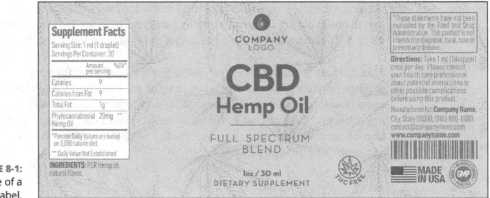

FIGURE 8-1:
An example of a typical CBD label.

Calin-H/Shutterstock.com

Although the potency of CBD may suggest an intended level of effectiveness, the form of the product also matters. Different forms are optimal for different functions, as I explain in Chapter 7. Additionally, bioavailability is higher for a sublingual than it is for an edible, for example, so a product potency described as a 30mg dose in a sublingual will have effects closer to 30mg, whereas an edible, because it has lower bioavailability, when it says its dose is 30mg, it is more like 10mg because edibles have lower bioavailability.

Edibles, sublinguals, topicals, and smokables all give different results. These various forms also have different onset times, so when they take effect and how long they last will be an added variable. So do different kinds of extracts like full-spectrum, broad-spectrum, distillate, or isolate.

And, to make it a bit more dynamic, as if it wasn't already, added complementary ingredients will not affect the potency but can affect the effectiveness of the feelings that may be associated with potency. For instance, should you choose a full-spectrum for pain, and it is made with curcumin or turmeric, you may feel an enhanced experience over just a straight full-spectrum.

Scheduling CBD into your daily routine

In my many years of practice and working with different individuals, I've found that the best way to incorporate anything new into your world is to find a way to stack it with an existing habit. If you can implement a new practice easily, you're more likely to stick with it because it feels complementary. Building a whole new routine can sometimes be harder to accomplish, which means potentially limited results. The following sections give three examples of ways to slot CBD into your normal day.

TIP

Onset times are important to factor in when you're dosing yourself. I break down onset times for various forms in Chapter 7, but in general, remember that smoking and inhalation are going to have the quickest onset time — between immediate and a few minutes. On the other end of the spectrum, edibles and capsules can take up to two hours depending on how full your stomach already is.

Dosing before bed

Do you sleep for as long or as deeply as you want? Maybe you need help getting to sleep or staying asleep. You may choose a specific form of CBD as part of your bedtime routine to help you achieve those desired results. For instance, if you have trouble falling asleep, incorporate an aid (specifically, an ingestible) into your routine before you go to bed. Carefully consider the form and the onset time of that particular product, whether it be a gummy or a tablet. If you find that you wake up in the night with pain, you can tweak your routine to optimize relief.

Perhaps you want to try a topical ointment right before you go to bed to increase the microcirculation and allow some time for absorption while you're sleeping.

Applying CBD after workouts

If you decide to use a CBD topical after a workout for muscle recovery, you need a game plan. The most effective move is to apply it directly after a shower, thus providing some moisture as well as potentially increasing the intended results. The ultimate idea of a CBD topical is that it gets into your system as efficiently as possible. Your body is warm and your heart rate is elevated when you work out, which allows for better circulation. The same is true after a hot shower.

Incorporating CBD at mealtimes

For supplemental purposes, or for addressing some conditions that require longer routines of CBD, mealtimes may be your best opportunity. Eating is necessary for survival, so if you're human, you get some sort of signal to eat and nourish your body. Cue the loud stomach growls! If you can find creative ways to incorporate your CBD into your mealtime routines, you can receive consistent benefits. Think about adding it to a smoothie or taking it with your other supplements in the morning before breakfast. You can even use a CBD olive oil in your salad dressing in the evening; the options are pretty much endless.

Realizing the importance of bioavailability

Bioavailability is just as important as onset time. *Bioavailability* is the amount of CBD that can enter into the body and bloodstream and is responsible for delivering the intended effects. Common theories suggest that 100 percent of the intended dose doesn't actually reach the bloodstream. For example, 30 percent bioavailability means that only 10 milligrams of a 30-milligram dose is available to your body. Table 8-1 shows the projected available dose of CBD that will access the bloodstream effectively based on form factor.

TABLE 8-1

Bioavailability of CBD by Form Factor

Form	Bioavailability
Inhalation	30%
Vaporization	Up to 50%
Sublingual	3–40%
Edibles	5–15%
Topical/transdermal	45%, noting that it's accessing a diversity of receptors

All the info in Table 8-1 is based on preliminary studies. Other factors that affect bioavailability include proper use of the products and the quality of the product's formulation.

Many manufacturers suggest that a particular product's bioavailability is increased in a water-soluble formulation (because the entire body is 60 percent water) or a nano-formulation (because it increases the surface area of the CBD molecule). Both are theories, like most of the "findings" in this space.

TIP

When choosing a product, keep in mind the following suggestions as they relate to potency and bioavailability:

>> Buy one that has the potency written clearly on the label, so you can trust the accountability of the brand.

>> Buy the form that is right based on what you will consume as you should based on your schedule.

>> Buy for a level of potency that considers the bioavailability of the form plus the required potency or higher — but not lower.

>> Buy the one that has the form that is best for the onset time and duration you require.

>> Adjust the dose of the product you take to your needs.

For example, say you're looking for a supplement dose of 10 milligrams, and you prefer a capsule. A capsule is 10 percent bioavailability, on average, so you would need to take a 100-milligram capsule. Alternately, if you were to take a sublingual with a supposed 30 percent bioavailability, you would need to take approximately a 33-milligram dose.

REMEMBER

Buying a potency that is higher than what you need (based on the ratio of bio-availability in Table 8-1) only makes sense if you are buying a straight CBD product because the products with other ingredients in them also scale in consumed volume when you dose up. For instance, an edible cookie might require that you eat five cookies, and you likely don't want or need all the other ingredients in the cookie in that high a volume. Similarly, for a pain product that also has active amounts of turmeric, when you dose up, you are also dosing up extra turmeric.

Keeping Others in Mind as You Dose in Public or at Work

What you do to eliminate your pain, manage your mood, or even soothe your anxiety is your business. Other than any required self-reporting, no one else really needs to know. With a few simple tips and tricks, you can use CBD discreetly when you're out and about. Professionalism and CBD use can easily coexist!

REMEMBER

Etiquette is etiquette, both in general and regarding cannabis specifically. If you're consuming something openly that may impact those around you, be considerate. Socially awkward moments are a reality, but good communication goes a long way. If you're comfortable with your activities, why you wouldn't inform and include those around you? Ask!

If you need to be discreet, do so. You have plenty of ways to avoid displaying your choices front and center, from choosing your consumption method wisely based on circumstances to politely removing yourself from a social or public setting to take care of your needs.

In particular, you may find that you need to use your CBD during the workday. People have been medicating at work for as long as you can imagine. Many employment contracts even have clauses about smoke breaks written in, so if your state allows it, who's to say you can't smoke CBD during those breaks as well as long as it doesn't affect your work?

TIP

My best advice in this situation is to determine whether your intended delivery form works for your business, your colleagues, and so on. For example, if you work at a post office, you likely can't vape your CBD as you accept incoming packages. But you may be able to wear a topical patch, or excuse yourself to the restroom to take a tincture under your tongue or put a mint in your mouth. Then carry on just like you would with any other mint or gum. Find a method of consumption that's sufficiently discreet so that you may not have to consider workplace ramifications. Flip to Chapter 7 for details on delivery methods.

Adjusting Your Usage to How Your Body Reacts

Little has been recorded about adverse reactions to CBD. This gap may be in part because CBD is such a new form of medicinal healing available in the marketplace at such a wide level. But really, research is starting to indicate it exists largely because there truly are few adverse reactions in general. To CBD itself, that is; you do also have to consider the other additives and ingredients in any given product.

WARNING

The main cause for concern is the liver. CBD is processed through your liver, so bad reactions from misuse and extra pharmaceuticals or liver-processed substances may create negative effects. Be sure to take your concerns to your doctor.

Looking at potential sleep reactions

Liver concerns aside, most would consider a "bad reaction" to be no reaction to the CBD at all. And if you're taking CBD as a supplement, sometimes you're better off not expecting a reaction as much as a compiled, long-term health opportunity.

Reactions are specific to your individual physiological makeup. The main two are

>> **A bit of drowsiness:** This reaction is the most common, though it still seldom happens. In really high doses, the effect can be a strong desire to sleep.

>> **Sleeplessness:** For some, CBD actually makes them a bit more sleepless, but this reaction is fairly uncommon.

If you find yourself drowsy, decrease your dose to see whether you can still get your intended benefits without the side effect. You can also simply dose yourself in the evening (or whatever time of day you sleep), when drowsiness is a benefit. On the other hand, if you find that CBD makes you a little restless and sleepless, try using it in the mornings so that you don't have a large concentration of it in your system when it's time for rest. If you follow the general recommendation to start slow and low with your dosing (see the following section), you can almost assuredly avoid these issues.

Finding the virtue in moderation: Microdosing

I tend to believe that all things are best in moderation — even, sometimes, moderation. In the case of CBD, slow and low is the best way to start out, particularly because you don't know your body or how it's going to react. You want to give it the best opportunity possible for success.

REMEMBER

Say it with me: slow and low.

The benefits of *microdosing* — consistently adding a concentration of a substance to your bloodstream so that you have a mild and gentle experience — can be significant over time. The whole fad of microdosing largely comes from psychedelic origins; it has seen a rise in popularity as an alternative to having some huge, mind-altering experience all at once that may be hard to integrate. Cannabis, because it can provide a psychedelic experience when it includes THC, has dominated the conversation of late.

In terms of incorporating CBD, looking for the benefits of microdosing may seem like a little bit of a lost conversation. Unlike with psychedelics, the idea of using CBD is to address a particular condition that may not necessarily be of mental origin.

TIP

Rather than *microdosing*, think about it more as *titrating* CBD, or starting with small amounts and gradually increasing as necessary in order to arrive at your intended effects. I cover titrating in Chapter 6.

Storing Your CBD Products

How you store your CBD matters, both for keeping it high-quality and for keeping it out of the wrong hands. The following sections explore a couple of storage considerations.

Preserving potency

Like anything else, CBD products have a shelf life, especially when you're talking about flower or something that doesn't come with an additional preservative to make it last longer. Products packed full of preservatives tend to have the longest shelf life. The idea of a preservative is to keep microbes or other bacterial contaminants from compromising the safety and, in some cases, the effectiveness of the product. That's why gas stations stock up on packaged pastries and not iceberg lettuce. Only one quickly wilts.

Because essentially no regulation covers what is or isn't in these products, you have to be on the lookout yourself. Product potency may not be compromised over the shorter term, but it can dwindle with time. Here are a few main causes of decreased CBD potency:

>> **Compromised other ingredients:** Even if the CBD in a product is fine, other ingredients may have become contaminated, making them unusable or otherwise unhealthy. Think of a jar of jam that's been sitting in the back of the

fridge for a year. You may find a healthy coating of mold skimming the top when you finally pop it open. Even if you don't actually see mold, the jam may be teeming with invisible microbial contaminants because it's been sitting for such a long period. The same can happen to products with CBD that may have been on the shelf at a local grocery store, gas station, or dispensary.

>> **Exposure to the elements:** You should handle anything you're buying carefully to protect it from potential contamination or degradation through air and light exposure. The important chemicals in CBD can become oxidized through exposure to air. These chemical compounds change over time, compromising not just their potency but also both their effects and their effectiveness.

REMEMBER

Many CBD tinctures are packaged in amber glass bottles to protect the product from harmful light degradation. Even with this layer of protection, don't store your tinctures in direct sunlight.

>> **Problematic packaging:** Over time, products packaged in plastic run the risk of incorporating other ingredients from the plastic itself that weren't necessarily a part of the initial formulation. For example, you've probably heard that a plastic water bottle sitting out in the sun can break down, contaminating your water with the plastic. The same goes for CBD products. Also keep in mind that shipping products around the country can expose them to hot and cold, again compromising the chemicals in the packaging.

So how can you maintain the potency of your CBD products? I'm glad you asked:

>> **Look for products that have an expiration date and are packaged in materials considerate of what's contained inside.**

>> **Store leftovers responsibly.** If it's a single-use product (like an edible) and you use only a portion do intend to finish it the next day.

>> **Be mindful of every aspect of your product, and expect the label to indicate that the manufacturer is too.**

>> **Keep it sanitary.** You don't have to surgically sterilize everything that comes in contact with your CBD, but you do want to avoid increasing its exposure to microbes and potentially reintroducing something from the outside into the product where you can. For example, you may want to scoop your topical out of the container with a (clean) spoon rather than, you know, your bare hand.

Some products will not have expiration dates. Without exception, each and every product should, but someone's always cutting corners. So if you find yourself with an open bottle of CBD tincture that's been sitting in the back of the drawer for six months prior, let it go. Assume it's no longer a spring chicken and get a new one. It may not be compromised, but the risks outweigh the benefits.

Restricting access

I've been in this industry long enough to see folks thinking they have the perfect hiding spot only to discover that kids and pets can be pretty clever (and doubly enticed by anything they see as a secret). That's why paying attention to where you stash your CBD is important.

Restricting access may seem like more of an issue for cannabis as a whole, but a certain amount of controversy still surrounds the effects, benefits, and legality of CBD. So until it's just an ingredient like any other on the back of a label, users need to make responsible decisions to protect these goods so that they don't accidentally fall into the hands of those who you may not want to get into it, may have adverse reactions, or may simply be too young to understand why these gummies aren't for kids.

Plenty of companies have built their businesses on creating bag sachets and lock-boxes to keep out those who don't have incredibly dexterous thumbs. Investing in one of these things may be worth your while. Know that the size of the satchel or lockbox may be better suited for a refrigerator or freezer rather than just a drawer.

3

Benefitting from CBD

Chapter **9**

Easing Neurological Conditions

C BD is an incredible tool to ease neurological conditions of various sorts. Some of the most pressing conditions and diseases that Western medicine has struggled to address are neurological. Historically speaking, symptom management was the default treatment for neurological conditions. This is because disease prevention or the slowing of the progression of the disease was an inaccessible option. Inflammation is being studied as the cause of many of these conditions; it also doubles as a side effect.

In this chapter, you explore inflammation from both angles and discover how CBD can be an ally. The conditions covered in this chapter, such as Huntington's, Alzheimer's, CFS (chronic fatigue syndrome), and MS (multiple sclerosis), are potential candidates for deeper research around cannabis remedies. Therefore, I also share with you some preliminary successes with CBD and future opportunities.

Acknowledging the Dangers of Inflammation and How CBD Can Help

Inflammatory conditions, or rather *chronic inflammatory diseases,* are one of the leading causes of death worldwide. And inflammation-related diseases contribute to an incredible amount of discomfort across the population. A whole host of things can cause inflammation, from *autoimmune diseases* (where your system mistakenly attacks healthy cells) to chemical irritants and intoxicants and even pollution.

Another contributor is oxidative stress. In the simplest terms, *oxidative stress* is caused by an imbalance between the production and accumulation of molecules responsible for signaling normal processes in cells. The result is that the body's detoxification system becomes impaired. This breakdown can ultimately lead to chronic inflammation.

Additionally, the inflammatory process can actually induce oxidative stress. Under normal circumstances, inflammation is a defense mechanism for combating infectious pathogens. However, uncontrolled inflammatory reactions worsen oxidative stress, compounding the problem. It's a vicious cycle.

Doing your homework on inflammatory conditions

Origin aside, inflammation is a big deal and not to be taken lightly. Research links chronic inflammation to diabetes, cancer, arthritis, heart disease, asthma, and even bowel diseases like Crohn's, celiac disease, and leaky gut. This kind of perpetual inflammation is gradual inflammation over long periods that inhibits bodily functions necessary for daily life. This gradual weakening of the immune system can be fatal.

One community of thought sees neurological diseases (Alzheimer's, Parkinson's, multiple sclerosis [MS], traumatic brain injuries, depression, autism, and more) as inflammation-centric. The most commonly encountered neurological conditions are chronic pain and anxiety, which affect up to half of adult Americans daily. If you have any connection to these whatsoever, you may understand how complicated they seem to be from a treatment standpoint in Western medical society. Questions about causes, treatment, and remediation plague both researchers and individuals looking to prevent these conditions.

Understanding CBD's anti-inflammatory and other neuroprotective properties

Early research suggests that CBD is highly anti-inflammatory, so no wonder it's being tried and tested across a variety of diseases. One important point is that CBD acts as a far-reaching anti-inflammatory after it's mobilized in the bloodstream. Ultimately, this means that even though you can't directly apply CBD to your brain, CBD in your bloodstream will still reach your brain.

This fact is significant for two reasons:

>> CB1 cannabinoid receptors, which are part of the body's internal cannabinoid or *endocannabinoid* system (ECS), are most prevalent in the brain.

>> CB2 receptors play a role in immune function.

CBD interacts with these receptors in your body, which has an impact on your body's reactions to internal and external events. I discuss the ECS in more detail in Chapter 3, but the takeaway here is that its main function lies in areas such as cognition, balance (homeostasis), motivation, emotional responses, and motor functions. That's why the implications for CBD as an anti-inflammatory are broad.

CBD's antioxidant properties can also be incredibly beneficial to the brain. Antioxidants inhibit the oxidization responsible for producing free radicals that lead to cell damage. This long-term cell damage is the root of chronic illness and disease.

Numerous studies have linked antioxidant-rich diets to reduced disease rates — everything from Parkinson's and Alzheimer's to arthritis to stroke and cardiovascular disease. Your body naturally produces antioxidants, but not on a high enough level to combat oxidative stress.

Beyond antioxidant properties, CBD has antifungal, antimicrobial, and antibacterial properties. This exhaustive span of properties may also combat some of the pathogens responsible for oxidative stress (theoretically, at least). When these properties work together, they can not only reduce the inflammation but also fight some of what's causing the inflammation. Clinical studies are already showing that CBD helps reduce damage to the brain and nervous system and encourages the growth and development of new neurons. By protecting against oxidative stress and improving recovery, CBD is a promising treatment for degenerative conditions.

Helping with Huntington's Disease

Huntington's disease is a rare and inherited condition that causes the perpetual breakdown of nerve cells essential to brain function. The results range from impaired cognitive function to psychiatric disorders and deteriorating movement.

Inflammation has been shown to increase the negative effects of Huntington's disease. Because of CBD's anti-inflammatory properties, theories and preliminary evidence suggest that it may help prevent further degeneration of Huntington's disease.

The following sections examine the various phases of Huntington's disease and some ways CBD may be able to treat some of the symptoms.

Looking at the five stages of Huntington's disease

Huntington's disease has five stages, but the names are straightforward:

>> Stage 1: Preclinical stage

>> Stage 2: The early stage

>> Stage 3: The middle stage

>> Stage 4: The late stage

>> Stage 5: The end-of-life stage

The life expectancy for someone with Huntington's can be between 10 and 20 years, and the variability in stages from patient to patient is dramatic. More often than not, only the first three stages are discussed because the latter two are largely about maintenance.

Stage one, preclinical, is when only mild symptoms are present and no doctor has diagnosed the condition. The average onset age of Huntington's patients is between 40 and 60, but it has come on as early as 2 and as late as 80 years old. During the preclinical stage, cognitive function isn't impaired, or at least doesn't require assistance, but the person may have an altered mood.

The second, early stage includes noticeable enough symptoms to begin to diagnose Huntington's disease. These symptoms include tremors in the outer extremities and sometimes nervous twitches and pain in the facial features. During the early stage, most people can do almost anything by themselves, including working and driving; however, sleeping and eating can be affected. The degenerative cognitive aspects appear as increased difficulty thinking and mood changes from irritability to depression to stress and anxiety.

By the middle stage (stage 3), the effects impact the person's ability to carry on most motor functions. People at this stage require substantial help and often 24-hour care to handle the most basic of chores. One of the most compromising motor functions is the difficulty swallowing, which may present a choking hazard. The psychological impacts can become more dominant at this stage because of the additional challenges (such as slurring speech and difficulty balancing and walking), resulting in full-blown depression.

In the late (fourth) stage, people require assistance in all areas of life and may be bedridden. Muscles seize and movements become rigid and slow — including in the facial features, which leads to speech impairment. The full inability to swallow by this point requires a feeding tube. Sleep and mood issues are only exacerbated at this point.

The end-of-life stage, stage five, is where the person becomes completely dependent and has only months to live. At this point, the best carers can do for them is to make them comfortable.

Improving quality of life

With a drug-resistant disease like Huntington's, researchers are continually on the search for new ways to help slow and even potentially prevent the disease. Many more studies still need to happen on a clinical level to determine whether CBD is a viable treatment for Huntington's disease. For example, can CBD delay the onset of new symptoms, or keep existing symptoms from worsening? The list goes on.

Recent clinical studies exploring how effective CBD is in minimizing the reduction of motor skills in people with Huntington's deemed it ineffective. Researchers tested low doses of CBD over six weeks against a placebo, and participants on the CBD showed no improvement. However, they also showed no side effects, and CBD at higher doses may be more effective.

Despite these results regarding mobility, the neuroprotective qualities of CBD are still promising as a remedy for the other uncomfortable symptoms of Huntington's. For example, CBD's success as an anti-inflammatory may be able to help keep the rest of the body functioning as highly as possible. The further degeneration of any other aspect of life seems like it's worth addressing, especially in the earlier stages of the disease.

CBD can also help treat additional symptoms of the disease, including stress, anxiety, and depression. Anecdotal evidence around remediating stress and anxiety with CBD has been really promising. Regular CBD doses of 10 to 50 milligrams a day, up to twice a day, may be a good starting point for people with Huntington's. The same supplemental dose may also help address the depression associated with advancing stages of the disease (see the preceding section).

Soothing Alzheimer's Disease

Alzheimer's disease is a neurodegenerative condition that represents the most common form of dementia. The disease begins with mild memory loss but evolves into a progressive and irreversible disorder. It slowly destroys the memory, along with thinking and reasoning skills. Eventually, the ability to perform any task is severely diminished. Late-onset Alzheimer's is the most common form, where adults in their 60s and beyond begin to experience symptoms.

Inflammation has been shown to increase the negative side effects and impacts of Alzheimer's disease, and CBD has been shown to offer inflammation relief. CBD may also reduce oxygen buildup and brain cell decline, all of which are part of degenerative diseases.

Analyzing inflammation of the brain

As I note earlier in the chapter, inflammation is the body's immune response to pathogens and bacteria throughout the system. It attacks not only the harmful pathogens but sometimes also the healthy brain cells. This immune response has been found to potentially contribute to the development of plaque and buildup in the brain that lead to Alzheimer's disease. In people with Alzheimer's, this immune response disproportionately attacks and damages healthy neurons, which in turn deepens the inflammatory response and results in further neurodegeneration.

Setting the stage for treatment

Although strong anecdotal evidence points to great potential, studies have only been done on mouse models to date. More evidence is available to suggest that CBD as a supplement may help with some of the other side effects of Alzheimer's and dementia: depression and agitated frustration. CBD's calming and soothing effects can help mitigate the emotional response. Strong and violent emotions are part of what makes this disease so uncomfortable.

Taking a regular daily supplemental dose of CBD may be a helpful tool for those experiencing Alzheimer's. At this stage, they likely take a plethora of prescribed medications, so adding a 10-to-30-milligram CBD gel cap or capsule form may be the easiest route.

I recommend a gel cap or capsule form because I acknowledge that adding something new to an Alzheimer's patient's routine may be complicated thanks to the memory loss. Finding a way to incorporate it into an established habit that's either managed by somebody else or so ingrained that it's not going away seems best.

TIP

You can find plenty such options on the market. Lean toward a full-spectrum product for the broadest possible benefit. (Flip to Chapter 7 for more on full-spectrum and other forms of CBD.) If you can find one with ginseng or ginkgo extract, which also support cognitive function, why not take advantage of the complementary and supportive herbs?

You can try a product by the brand Wildflower, which is a capsule with ginseng, curcumin, and 20 milligrams of CBD. Plant People brand also has a product called Stay Sharp in a capsule form for cognitive function.

Tackling Chronic Fatigue Syndrome (CFS)

Yet another medically unexplainable disease, chronic fatigue syndrome (CFS), is left untreated because so little is known. CFS has an almost endless list of symptoms, including unexplained muscle and joint pain, dizziness headaches, sore throats, brain fog, enlarged lymph nodes, and restless sleep. For the most part, dealing with the disease is about managing the symptoms, many of which CBD may relieve.

Making sense of the symptoms

Chronic fatigue syndrome is characterized by

>> Extreme fatigue that lasts six months or more

>> Symptoms that seem to worsen with any physical or mental exertion and don't seem to improve with rest

>> A feeling of chronic pain

>> Unrefreshing sleep, chronic insomnia, or other sleep disorders

>> Memory loss, difficulty concentrating, and faintness

These incredibly diverse symptoms don't really make sense together, and that may be why Western medicine has found itself so stumped. Treating such a variety of symptoms pharmacologically can result in a whole other set of side effects that may not be much better than some of the symptoms themselves.

Fighting a two-headed dragon: Pain and inflammation

REMEMBER

The official cause of CFS is unknown, but the speculation is that it may be caused by viruses, a weakened immune system, hormonal imbalances, and stress. CFS most affects women, starting in their 40s and 50s. The other imbalances women experience at that stage in their lives may also potentially play a part.

Because so many CFS symptoms show up across the entire body and immune system, inflammation is undoubtedly a piece of the CFS puzzle. The pain associated with CFS is a not a symptom of physical trauma, per se, so inflammation is likely partially to blame here as well. As I write this, the newest and most promising study to the CFS table is by the Stanford University School of Medicine. It indicates a new link to molecules within the body that are responsible for signaling cells for immune function and reactions to inflammation and infection.

A breakdown in cell signaling may lead to an increase in inflammation, creating a cycle and possibly compromising healthy tissue in the process. This compromise degrades healthy cells and affects how the body reacts with swelling, redness, and pain. (If this faulty cell signaling sounds like the oxidative stress I discuss earlier in the chapter, it should. Head to the earlier section "Acknowledging the Dangers of Inflammation and How CBD Can Help" for more on that topic.)

Treating CFS symptoms with CBD

Whether CBD can treat the root cause of chronic fatigue syndrome is unclear (especially because no one is sure what that root cause is; see the preceding section). But a daily CBD supplement may offer a little bit of relief from some of the symptoms. For example, CBD can help treat sleep conditions and chronic pain, both of which are often associated with CFS (see the earlier section "Making sense of the symptoms"). You can read more about CBD's effects on these and other pillars of CBD relief in Chapter 5.

TIP

Start with a supplemental dose of ten milligrams twice a day for three days. You can adjust the dose from there as I describe in Chapter 6 if you're not experiencing results. The best form is the one that makes you feel best. Make it easy for yourself.

If you find yourself experiencing different, deepened CFS symptoms at various times throughout the day or week, having another dose or form of CBD around may be helpful. Layering on an extra dose when the symptoms occur may help mitigate them.

REMEMBER

For symptoms that come on quickly, like migraines or localized pain, a fast-acting smokable, tincture, or mint is the best bet.

Addressing the Symptoms of Multiple Sclerosis (MS)

Multiple sclerosis (MS) is an unpredictable and debilitating disease of the central nervous system. Dysfunction in the immune system causes the body to attack the nerve fibers, which disrupts the flow of communication between the brain and the body. MS largely affects the brain, the spinal cord, and the optic nerves, and its progression is devastating.

Describing the disease and its symptoms

MS has no known cause, but it's classified as an autoimmune disease. The wide range of symptoms includes the following:

>> Extreme tiredness

>> Blurry vision/total loss of sight

>> Severe pain

>> Changes in sensation throughout the entire body, like tingling or numbness

>> Difficulty walking and balancing, which may lead to falls and even becoming wheelchair-bound

Though MS isn't considered fatal, life expectancy for someone with this disease is usually five to ten years shorter than that of the average adult. Complications such as infections may further compromise the body and potential life expectancy.

Supporting your nervous system

When the covering on nerve fibers is compromised in an MS attack, the body's reactions range from tingling sensations to fatigue, pain, and weakness. This effect is not only stressful but also debilitating.

Stress has long been considered a potential factor in the onset and further aggravation of MS. Stress on the body and mind sends the nervous system into a "fight or flight" response, producing high levels of the stress hormones, cortisol and adrenalin. When this response happens, the body shifts its energy into fighting off the threat. Stress further compromises your immune response. From my personal experience and anecdotal evidence, addressing the stress response may be one of the most important things to improve quality of life both mentally and physiologically for people with MS.

Further research is necessary, but CBD has also been indicated to protect the immune system and thus may play a role in autoimmune conditions. If a simple CBD regimen can help reduce the feeling of stress and maybe in turn the immune response to stress, people with MS may be able to get some relief. All these areas of study around CBD are promising for MS patients.

Here, as with any other disease of the nervous system, consider adding a dose of CBD to your existing regimen, as long as that regimen doesn't already contain a high concentration of other medications your liver has to process. Start low and slow with ten milligrams twice a day in whatever form feels best and see whether you can find some relief. You can then up the dose as necessary (see Chapter 6).

REMEMBER

Very severe cases and really intense symptoms of MS may call for high doses. If you find yourself reaching doses in the 100-to-200-milligram range, make sure to double-check with your MS specialist for any contraindications related to liver function.

Resolving and reducing the symptoms

Beyond supplementation, here are a few other options for potentially relieving some of the symptoms of MS with CBD:

>> **Vaping:** A vape pen may be a really great way to alleviate MS attacks. Pens containing high concentrations of CBD, along with very mild concentrations of THC, may offer full-body relaxation and also alleviate a bit of stress. The brain remembers when it experiences pain or uncomfortable sensations repeatedly over years. The CBD may treat the pain in the short term, but your system continues to tell your brain that the pain is there. I mention THC specifically here because it's what helps your brain break out of the pattern. You can read about vaping in Chapter 7; Chapter 6 has details on the legality of THC in various U.S. states.

TIP

Baths: If your MS attacks result in more residual, longer-lasting sensations, from tingling and numbness to cramps and tightness, hop in a bathtub with a CBD bath soak or bath bomb. They're super relaxing and contain high concentrations of CBD for ultimate relief. Choose a soak with at least a cup of Epsom salt if you suffer from muscle cramping; otherwise, a bath bomb should do the trick. Either of these options should have at least 50 milligrams of CBD per bath, and up to 150 milligrams for maximum effectiveness. Verte Essentials, Vertly, Empower, and Papa & Barkley are all great brands, easily available online or at www.shop-poplar.com. I am the Co-Founder and Chief Product Officer at Poplar, which means I am responsible for selecting every single product that touches our shelves. I am confident that the brands we carry can back their products with integrity and efficacy, so I feel comfortable making those recommendations to you.

>> **Topicals:** If a CBD bath sounds intimidating and you don't want to take something internally, topicals are another option. CBD topicals, while not as effective for inflammation or immune system support, can be helpful for regional pain and MS attacks.

Inevitably, changes in the spine and nerve damage cause discomfort. A good balm, salve, or lotion with complementary ingredients like arnica, comfrey, calendula, and magnesium is going to provide much-needed relief. I cover topicals in more detail in Chapter 7. Because of compromised mobility, and discomfort in mobility, companies like Apothecanna have created a spray-on pain relief product that dries in place and is really easy to apply. They also have other widely available products great for pain. Bade Collection makes a really nice topical balm with CBD as well and offers movement instruction for relieving pain in tired muscles.

>> **CBD plus THC:** The combination of THC and CBD in a 1:1 ratio is beginning to open doors. Early clinical research indicates that this combination specifically can reduce muscle spasticity and associated pain. *Spasticity* is the tightening of muscles that then resist being stretched.

Although they haven't been studied yet as MS treatments extensively, some other avenues may be promising. The FDA has approved the synthetic CBD drug Epidiolex for epilepsy, a condition that also results in muscle spasticity. It may therefore have implications for MS. Maybe a host of other plant medicines, such as chamomile, which is known to help with muscle spasms and is anti-inflammatory, or arnica, in combination with CBD will help because they are so good at supporting muscle relaxation.

Chapter 10

Alleviating Autoimmune Conditions

A n *autoimmune disease* is a condition where your immune system mistakenly attacks itself. The immune system protects you from invasive germs that include bacteria and viruses, sending out protective cells as a reaction to ward off them off. Through some malfunction, an autoimmune condition triggers your system when no threat is actually there. On high alert, your immune system harms and attacks healthy cells. No hard evidence suggests why this misfire happens, but some schools of thought link it to inflammation.

All studies point to the fact that CBD protects the immune system and plays a role in quelling autoimmune conditions. Throughout this chapter, I cover some of the potential benefits of CBD and its fellow plant molecules as immune supports.

Understanding CBD and Immune Function

The immune system is a complex network of cells and proteins programmed to protect the body against unknown microbes. The proper functioning of an immune system means that cells actively fight off disease and infection.

A compromised immune system can be the result of outside invaders, but internal enemies like stress and autoimmunity can hit you with friendly fire. Inflammation is how your body defends itself against those outside invaders. CBD is an anti-inflammatory, so ultimately it also regulates and protects the immune system.

Connecting cannabis and autoimmunity

It all sounds simple: Immunity is when good cells balance the body. Autoimmune diseases cause good cells to attack good cells. CBD protects the immune system.

Sorry to disappoint, but it's much more complicated than that. Both CBD's interaction with the immune system and the cells involved in these immune responses are diverse. And how they interact with one another varies widely. For this reason (and a few others), research in this area still has a long way to go.

Inflammation

The two most significant links here are the immune-protecting and anti-inflammatory capabilities of CBD. Treatment and therapy for autoimmune diseases isn't exhaustive, and frequently the root cause for the patient is left unidentified, so doctors are left to treat exclusively the symptoms. One of the immune dysfunction side effects of an attack on healthy cells is an inflammation response, so anti-inflammatory medications are helpful. CBD as an anti-inflammatory can help mediate that response and can act as a protective agent.

REMEMBER

Inflammation is one of the most critical processes in the immune system, if not *the* most critical. CBD's anti-inflammatory properties are technically as an *immune suppressant* and as *immunomodulators*. Translation: CBD can remediate an unruly and out-of-control immune response.

Stress

As with any debilitating disease, stress is a factor in autoimmune disease. A Harvard study suggests that stress may cause autoimmune disorders such as lupus, psoriasis, celiac disease, and rheumatoid arthritis. It found that autoimmune diseases were more prevalent among those previously diagnosed with stress-related disorders. It suggests that a peak stress event triggers the onset of an immune disease and that stress can exacerbate the symptoms of someone already exhibiting characteristics of such a disease. CBD is worth exploring as a remedy for anxiety and stress factors in the body.

A HISTORY OF SELF-MEDICATION

Patients have been self-medicating with cannabis for years. HIV makes the body more susceptible to common autoimmune diseases, often resulting in AIDS. This community was treating itself through cannabis community centers as early as the 1980s.

Tackling terpenes

As I discuss in Chapter 2, *terpenes* are plant chemicals with a lot of jobs, including protection, regeneration, recovery, and overall immunity. They're also responsible for the aroma and flavor of plants. Terpenes are essential to plant medicine. For millennia, people have been using them and their complementary properties to heal the human body.

Terpenes became a hot topic in the cannabis space because of their high concentrations in cannabis plants. But they're also part of the aromatherapy conversation because terpenes are also present in essential oils; essential oils are extracts of all the various terpenes in — you guessed it — an oil format.

Following is a list of the more common terpenes with anti-inflammatory benefits, along with their other services. They exist in the food you eat and serve as complementary ingredients in botanical medicines.

>> **Limonene** is one of the more common and recognizable terpenes. As the name suggests, it appears in citrus fruits' rinds and is responsible for their distinct citrusy scent. Its chemical properties are antiviral, antidiabetic, antioxidant, antidepressant, and antianxiety. It also plays a role in immune cell behavior and can help with gastric reflux.

>> **Beta-caryophyllene,** one of my favorites, exists in higher concentrations in black pepper and cloves than in anything else. It has a bright, earthy, and spicy scent. Like CBD, no evidence has linked this terpene to addiction or tolerance development. This makes it a strong contender as a pain reliever for those suffering from long-term and chronic pain.

>> **Linalool** is a dominant terpene in the lavender plant, but it's also present in birch, rosewood, and citrus. It creates a rich and forward scent that's quite polarizing. Some associate it with calmness and relaxation. Linalool is useful for insomnia and convulsions. Its chemical properties are antianxiety, anti-cancer, antidepressant, neuroprotective, and antimicrobial.

>> **Humulene** is quite prevalent in hops and coriander, but you can also find it in ginger and cloves. It has an earthy and woody scent. It can reduce allergic

reactions in the airways and is promising in asthma research, though it's not a bronchodilator. Known as an antibacterial and pain reliever, it's also suggested to be a protective agent in cells and an appetite suppressant.

>> **Pinene** is (unsurprisingly) abundant in pine needles, but you also find it across various freshly scented plants and herbs like rosemary and basil. It affects neurological stimulation for memory, attention, and alertness and also helps bronchial dilation.

>> **Myrcene,** found in hops, mango, lemongrass, and thyme, is also quite prevalent in cannabis. Soothing and relaxing by nature, it has a musky, sharp, and herbaceous scent. It's said to be neuroprotective and can protect the brain from oxidative damage in very high doses. (Chapter 9 has more on oxidative damage.)

TIP

When you're consuming cannabis, you want to look for a full- or broad-spectrum product (see Chapter 7) with a list of terpenes on the certificate of authenticity (COA; see Chapter 6). Complementary ingredients in your products can also work with the terpene profiles to support the effects you're trying to get.

Comparing CBD to conventional treatments

Traditionally, treatment for those with autoimmune diseases often involves medications designed to reduce inflammation and calm down the body's immune response. Other treatments include immunosuppressive drugs, which (as the name suggests) suppress the immune system or simply shut it off. The results are body-wide, as opposed to localized and symptom-specific. Some immunosuppressants come with a host of nasty side effects because of the compromises to your immune system. These drugs are, however, considered the gold standard.

Natural remedies for autoimmune diseases mainly consist of recommendations to reduce stress. That's not to say that people aren't finding plenty of other treatments for their symptoms, but, as a whole, the diseases have been quite hard to treat.

Given CBD's immune-supporting abilities, its future exploration (along with cannabis) as a remedy for autoimmune disease seems probable. To date, some studies are likely underway, but as with most areas of cannabis research in specific conditions, this field is in its infancy. The best opportunity seems to come from CBD's system-wide anti-inflammatory properties. Considering current treatments for autoimmune diseases lean heavily on anti-inflammatories, this is an excellent one-to-one comparison. It then becomes about finding the right form and dose to achieve the desired level of relief. The intended outcome would be a systematic reduction in inflammation and potential pain relief.

Another opportunity is to look at CBD as a stress reliever. Stress relief and relaxation are common recommendations to people with autoimmune diseases to prevent attacks on the system and potentially improve their overall experiences with their conditions.

REMEMBER

A glimmer of hope: CBD's potential to repair oxidative stress implies possible recovery from current damages. Additionally, early research has indicated that CBD may suppress the immune system's "memory," meaning the potential to cut down on future autoimmune attacks is there.

Relieving Lupus Symptoms

Lupus is an autoimmune disease that can cause inflammation and pain throughout the entire body. A combination of genetic and environmental factors likely triggers the onset of the disease, although the ultimate cause is unknown.

Like in many autoimmune conditions, system-wide inflammation and pain are significant concerns for people with lupus. CBD has a couple of potential applications here:

>> It functions as an anti-inflammatory and pain reliever.

>> It doesn't have the same dependency implications as many pharmaceuticals, so it's an excellent option because sustaining high doses of medicine for prolonged periods may be necessary in lupus treatment.

This section provides a quick overview of lupus symptoms and how CBD might help.

EXAMINING YOUR FAMILY TREE

Lupus is more likely to affect women of color than white women and is a condition that celebrities such as Toni Braxton and Selena Gomez grapple with. One of my friends recently found out that her grandmother has lupus. This discovery prompted her to do some research, and she found that African American women such as her are not only more likely to have lupus but also more likely to go undiagnosed and develop life-threatening complications. (One in 250 Black women will contract lupus in their lifetime.) Looking into your family history is worthwhile — regardless of whether you're a woman of color — to know whether this disease is present in your bloodline or extended family tree.

Addressing the effects of lupus

Lupus can come on as early as the teens and into the 30s. Because of flare-ups, early presentations of lupus can be challenging to detect. Initial signs of lupus can include the following:

>> Joint pain and fatigue

>> Fever

>> Weight changes

>> Gastrointestinal (GI) problems

>> Thyroid issues

>> Kidney challenges

>> Hair loss

>> Dry eyes and mouth

Some people have persistent and chronic lupus with frequent flare-ups, while others experience less frequency; the disease may even go into remission. Often, clinical tests can detect issues like excessive protein in the urine and blood imbalances like excessive antibodies and low blood cell counts.

The symptoms of lupus range from skin irritations and sensitivities all the way to inflammation and nerve problems. The following list delves into some of these symptoms. Not every symptom is present in all lupus cases, but even just a handful of these is plenty.

>> **Skin issues:** The skin irritation appears as a butterfly-shaped rash on the nose or cheeks and/or inflamed patches of skin. Ulcers can appear in the nose or mouth. Other problems can include increased sensitivity to light and sun or flaky, scaly, purplish-red spots on the outer extremities and face.

>> **Inflammation:** The severe inflammation and pain associated with lupus often compromise basic human function. Inflammation can appear in the lining of the heart or the lungs and contribute to arthritis in potentially two or more joints. Inflammation in the kidneys can make filtering toxins and waste from the blood — the kidneys' primary function — challenging. Indicators of kidney dysfunction include swelling in the lower extremities, increased blood pressure, bloody or dark urine, and localized kidney pain. Inflammation in the lungs can create breathing issues by compromising the muscles and shrinking the lung capacity.

>> **GI and thyroid problems:** Gastrointestinal problems can create heartburn and acid reflux, among other things. The thyroid, which is responsible for controlling the body's metabolism, can cause weight gain or loss. It can also have different effects on vital organs, with minor symptoms such as dry hair and skin and moodiness. This symptom alone is a separate condition entirely; depending on the symptoms, it's either *hypothyroidism* (an underactive thyroid) or *hyperthyroidism* (an overactive thyroid).

>> **Dryness:** Dryness in the mouth and the eyes can be an additional development called Sjögren's syndrome that affects the glands that produce moisture (such as tears and saliva). Women may also experience a dry vagina.

>> **Nerve issues:** Nerve problems can vary and sometimes include seizures. Nerve effects from lupus present in the peripheral nervous system, which is responsible for sensations and motor responses. The impact on these nerves from a lupus flare-up can range from numbness and tingling, much like in multiple sclerosis (MS), to limited mobility, like in Huntington's disease. You can read more about these and other neurological conditions in Chapter 9.

How much lupus may attack the peripheral nervous system, resulting in inflammation and potentially chronic pain, is still unclear.

>> **Liver and kidney problems:** Both liver and kidney problems can present with lower extremity swelling, dark urine, hair loss, and fatigue.

>> **Other symptoms:** Other symptoms of lupus include muscle and chest pain, osteoporosis, and depression. On rare occasions, anemia, seizures, and dizziness may appear.

Treating lupus-related skin conditions with CBD

Most people suffering from lupus are going to experience some sort of skin complications. As I mention in the preceding section, the primary skin conditions associated with lupus are the telltale butterfly–shaped rash, increased light/sun sensitivity, and flaky, scaly spots.

CBD to the rescue! Skin health is one of the pillars of CBD relief (see Chapter 5). Topicals may be an unlikely option for those with limited mobility and severe pain, but regular ingestibles in pill or tincture form are worth a try. The following sections discuss internal and external treatment for skin issues in lupus. You can read more about the various delivery methods for CBD in Chapter 7.

Because people with lupus are likely on some form of prescription medication, making sure they have no contraindications that may affect delivery of prescribed medication is important. For more on the how and why of drug interactions with CBD, refer to Chapter 5. It's extremely crucial for those who have lupus to pay particular note because CBD and other drug interactions affect the liver, and lupus patients can already have liver and/or kidney disfunction from the disease that would manifest similar symptoms.

Internally

Skin symptoms of the disease, as well as general discomforts, are exacerbated internally. So addressing lupus internally with CBD may help alleviate some of the topical signs of lupus. That's not to say exploring topical applications of CBD isn't helpful, just that pairing them with internal use may be most beneficial.

In exploring opportunities for internal consumption, it's best to consider the process a systemic approach to inflammation — where doses are designed to be taken regularly at intervals — keeping a concentration of CBD in the system all the time. For this reason, onset time and duration are less of a consideration, but because you would be taking it so frequently, a form that you appreciate taking is likely the best option. Sublinguals may be preferable for their ease, consistency, and bioavailability. The volume of your dose will be relative to the severity of your symptoms, and it may be a bit of a process coming to find the right dose. Starting with a supplemental dose, I might explore a 20-milligram dose two times a day to start, again being wary of what might appear as a liver or kidney reaction. If, after three days, you start to experience relief, you might back off the dose by 10 milligrams and see if you still feel relief. If so, you are getting closer to the right dose for you. Alternately, if you need to dose up, do it in three-day increments.

You will not build up a tolerance to CBD, so once you find your dose, there you may stay. Also note that if you should find relief and are using it for several months, and then you stop using it, your body may still feel relieved for a period of time, even a few months, where everything in your system feels in balance. However, the symptoms may come back as that supplement balance readjusts back to where it was before. So, the point is, if it's working, trust it.

Externally

Steroids are the traditional topical treatment for lupus. The steroids are contained in a cream or a gel form, and sometimes they do the job of relieving the topical flare-ups. Sun exposure almost always amplifies any sort of skin flare-up, so using sunscreen should be at the top of the list for helping prevent flare-ups.

Some CBD sunscreens are starting to hit the market, but they're in their infancies. I've tried only one, and my one-word review is "yikes." It almost instantly gave me a rash, so for now, keep your eyes peeled as CBD skincare evolves in both accessibility and formulation.

Prolonged treatment with steroid creams and gels can have nasty side effects such as thinner skin and enlarged hair follicles. You also may end up in a worse place than where you started. The purpose of a topical steroid is to reduce inflammation.

In my experience, topical CBD in the proper amounts can significantly reduce redness, inflammation, and swelling. I haven't personally seen it used to treat lupus, but I have seen it in action with other topical flare-ups. CBD interacts with inflammation topically and internally. It isn't necessarily interacting with the *endocannabinoid system when applied topically* (your body's internal cannabinoid system; see Chapter 3), but it does interact with a bunch of other topical receptors.

Choose a topical that you know won't exacerbate symptoms. If you've had any reaction to any skin creams, lotions, or oils in the past, be wary of those ingredients in your CBD products as well. You don't want to give your body any more work. Plenty of different forms are explicitly designed for ease of use. And though the heavier forms (like balms or salves) are better for pain relief, traditional lotions or water-based topicals may be a little bit better for skin rashes and irritations.

Here are a couple of product recommendations:

>> Empower Bodycare makes some great high-concentration CBD lotions. They were designed with pain and inflammation in mind. This form, which is a combination of oil-base and water-base, may be the easiest to apply and have a high enough concentration for the toughest of skin irritations. Empower sells directly on its website (www.empowerbodycare.com) and is available at my online multi-brand store, Poplar (www.shop-poplar.com), as well as many other retailers.

>> Women experiencing vaginal dryness should consider Quim, a cool product line, designed specifically for women, that contains a moisturizer. With the CBD craze, many brands are coming to the market with general remedies in mind, so finding products designed with a particular function in mind, like Quim's, is great. It's available in Quim's web store online (www.itsquim.com), and also on Poplar.

Treating the Effects of Lyme Disease

Lyme disease, contracted from the bite of infected black-legged ticks, has been reported in the 48 contiguous U.S. states as well as Alaska. However, the majority of infections are still focused in the Midwest and the Northeast. Since the 1990s, reported cases have gone up significantly in the Northeast.

The disease can affect anyone as long as a tick bites them. Hiking, golfing, camping, hanging around grassy and forested environments — when people play where ticks play, they're rolling the dice.

Lyme disease presents various symptoms:

>> General long-lasting fatigue (the major complaint)

>> Fever and headaches

>> A circular red rash when the disease is initially contracted

>> Arthritis

>> Facial paralysis

CBD can undoubtedly be a friend to those experiencing symptoms of this disease, as I explain in the following sections.

Looking at how CBD can help ease general symptoms of Lyme disease

TIP

If you've been bitten, fine-tune your eyes for the clear signs of Lyme. The indicative bull's-eye rash of Lyme and accompanying muscle and joint aches may not show up for several days or weeks after the tick bite. And even then, only 70 to 80 percent of people get a rash. Positive tests and Lyme disease cases can often be treated in the early stages with a few weeks of antibiotics. If you don't catch it in time, its complications and symptoms are beyond tedious. (Prevention is the best treatment, as I explain in the nearby sidebar.)

CBD can't make your time in the outdoors safer from ticks, but it certainly has the right properties to treat the side effects of Lyme disease. Reducing headaches, relieving nausea, and strengthening the immune system are crucial pieces to the symptomatic puzzle that CBD can ultimately address. Other possible symptoms of Lyme disease, such as nerve issues, pain episodes, anxiety, and depression, are also reported to be in the CBD wheelhouse.

THE BEST TREATMENT FOR LYME IS PREVENTION

If you identify as outdoorsy, be vigilant and plan ahead.

Be mindful of the seasons when tick activity is most prevalent. Most cases of the disease are reported in late spring and early summer.

Keep in mind that the window before Lyme disease detection is possible in the blood is about six weeks. You have approximately 36 hours after the tick bites you before you contract the disease, giving you more than an entire day to find a tick attached to your skin.

I've been bitten by ticks before because I tend to spend a lot of time outdoors. It's not pretty, I promise you. When you're spending time outside running around in the weeds, check your body head to toe for these little guys. They can be tiny, only swelling up to a noticeable size when they're full of your blood. Check your pets, too. They're more likely to track ticks indoors with all that fur.

A bite isn't pleasant, but removing ticks is even worse. The longer they're on your body, the deeper they burrow their heads into your skin, making them harder to remove. A few tick removal methods exist. One mentions burning the back of the tick with a blown-out match so that it backs out of your skin, but I think the universally preferred method is pinching the tick at the base of the neck with tweezers and slowly and gently removing it to be sure you remove every piece of its body.

Diminishing diarrheas and intestinal problems

An unpleasant side effect of Lyme disease is the toll that it takes on the intestinal tract. Children and adolescents more often experience these symptoms, but adults can get them, too. Abdominal pain, heartburn, vomiting, diarrhea, nausea, and sometimes even blood in the stool are byproducts. Many of these symptoms can be attributed to inflammation in the GI tract.

CBD alleviates the GI issues that result from gut inflammation, so it may well have benefits for Lyme disease as well. Because these symptoms are more common in children, I'm going to direct you to some of the CBD treats that may be more appealing for the young ones. When you're trying to incorporate something into a regular routine for a child, it has to have more appeal than a capsule. Luckily, the CBD market is full of gummies. And when I say full, I mean quite literally saturated. In every direction you look, you're going to find some form of a gummy, whether it's shaped like a bear or a square, for the young and the young at heart.

TIP

Look for gummies with the highest quality ingredients. Highline Wellness is a brand that has a variety of flavors. It has a combination of all-natural, high-quality ingredients that's unparalleled. Additionally, its Rest and Digest formula is made with apple cider vinegar, a natural digestive aid, making it a perfect complement to gastrointestinal issues.

Mints are another excellent option, and Mr. Moxey's mints are one of my favorites. The Relief mint has ginger, which soothes the stomach and relieves nausea. They're great for sucking on and come in low doses, so you can take them multiple times throughout the day to relieve effects.

Supplementing to address pain and muscle spasms

The pain relieving and anti-inflammatory properties of CBD can provide great assistance with the widespread muscle aches, pains, and spasms that come with Lyme disease. As with many autoimmune conditions, inflammation may be at the core. Taking CBD internally as a daily supplement is a good place to start. Any form will do here, but I like to start with a tincture because they have a quick onset and calculating the dosage is easy. You have so many products with complementary ingredients to choose from.

TIP

2Rise makes a potent tincture with turmeric as a complementary ingredient, making it one of my go-to's for inflammation and pain relief. If the pain is intense, Lily brand has a higher concentration of full-spectrum that I like. Follow the clear user directions on the bottles.

Generally speaking, start with a single dose in the morning and see whether that provides relief. I almost always suggest another dose by late afternoon and into the evening because the days are long and a lot of people still have to power through the night. If you're not finding relief from these two doses a day after three days, dose up by 5 milligrams and repeat for another three days. (As I explain in Chapter 6, CBD takes about a three-day window for CBD to get into your system and help you find a little bit of balance.)

TIP

If you need instant relief for any GI issues, feel free to layer in those gummies or mints in the preceding section. For any acute-onset pain, try an inhalation method; for regional pain, have a topical around. If all these internals sound like too much, create a stash of transdermal patches so you can try the same systematic three-day approach to getting CBD into your system.

Finding Help for Celiac Disease

Celiac disease is an autoimmune disease characterized by damage in the small intestine from ingesting gluten. It can come on anytime, and stress may cause or trigger a reaction. Those with a parent, sibling, or extended family member who has the disease have a higher chance of developing it. For some, celiac is mild enough that it goes untreated for many years. For others, it's so peculiar in its severity that it can go unrecognized. People suffering from other autoimmune diseases can also be subject to celiac.

Generally speaking, those diagnosed with celiac can curtail the symptoms and get back on track to feeling well again. During the process of getting well, CBD can be an ally; when you're feeling all good, you may no longer need it. This section covers the basics of celiac disease and how CBD can help treat its various symptoms.

REMEMBER

The only way to treat celiac disease itself is to remove gluten from your diet permanently.

Familiarizing yourself with the symptoms

The symptoms of celiac disease are quite similar to broader GI disorders:

>> Diarrhea or constipation

>> Bloating and gas

>> Nausea

>> Vomiting

>> Abdominal pain

>> Weight loss

>> Fatigue

Most of these symptoms relate specifically to GI and digestive issues, but beyond that, the list is long:

>> Weak and brittle bones, joint pain, and stiffness (because celiac hampers the small intestine's ability to take in nutrients)

>> Numbness and tingling associated with peripheral nerve pain in the hands and the feet

>> Reproductive issues such as irregular menstruation, miscarriage, and even infertility

>> Skin disorders

>> Seizures

Pinpointing possible gluten in CBD products

About anything gluten-free these days has a stamp on the side of the jar or the box proclaiming its gluten-freedom. That doesn't seem to extend to the CBD space yet, but it's only a matter of time as the CBD product market expands more and more into food.

REMEMBER

As you dip your toe into CBD, your best bet may be just to avoid all the snacky treats — cookies, crackers, candies, cakes, pies — and even the CBD beers (yes, CBD beer is a thing). Otherwise, be sure you understand which ingredients don't contain gluten.

CBD oil itself, as an infusion or extract from the plant with no other additives than the oil, should be gluten-free. *However,* do your research. Some oils may be made in facilities that produce another CBD product that does contain gluten; many brands across the entire CBD market are made within the same facilities. Some of the larger brands own their facilities, which makes spotting potential contaminants in the factory easier. Similarly, some of the super tiny brands do their own production and have the same kind of control.

Pairing widespread and specific CBD treatment for celiac relief

The broadest benefit from CBD for celiac disease is going to be a system-wide approach coupled with a regional approach. System-wide CBD concentrations and supplemental forms, taken regularly, can help get the body back to a state of balance. Address the symptoms specifically as needed, with ginger-infused CBD mints for nausea, turmeric and CBD beverages for GI repair (see the following section), and skin-focused CBD oils for topical manifestations.

Managing intestinal issues with CBD

Managing the intestinal issues is without a doubt the most critical piece of treating celiac symptoms. Your small intestine likely took a degree of damage before you got a diagnosis, so some reparative work is in order.

Much of the damage to the intestinal walls of your GI tract is going to result in inflammation. For maximum effectiveness, you want to address the GI tract from inside with a supplemental form of CBD to filter into the bloodstream and address system-wide inflammation. You can also try particular types of CBD in and through your small intestine. On an empty stomach, explore beverages containing doses of CBD. Choose something as natural and calming as possible. The fewer ingredients, the better.

TIP

Buddha Teas has a caffeine-free turmeric blend tea with a winning combination of anti-inflammatory turmeric to complement the CBD and ginger to soothe the stomach. Glow Water brand has a selection of teas that are available on its website that look nice, though I haven't tried them. The Sleep tea has complementary soothing ingredients. Take it right before bed and at least two hours after a light meal. Other beverage options are packets of drink mix; I suggest adding them to hot or warm water to decrease the amount of work your body has to do to absorb and work with the mixture. Prima makes some lovely, trustworthy blends. Steer clear of the sugar-packed mixes because refined sugar just complicates digestion and increases inflammation.

REMEMBER

Though CBD can help address the inflammation in the gut from a celiac reaction, avoiding gluten is always best for people with celiac.

Chapter **11**

Dealing with Eating Disorders and Digestive Troubles

Digestive and eating disorders, at their core, are all about nutrient uptake. These nutrients are paramount for normal life processes and functionality. Without them, your body struggles not only to find energy but also to support other vital functions like hormone balance, immune function, stress management, and more.

Eating disorders are in a category of their own because they have the stigma of just being about food control. But beyond that general and limited view, eating disorders negatively impact health and emotions as well. They're actually quite severe conditions and, left unaddressed, can be fatal.

In this chapter, I cover a range of conditions that require healing the digestive system and addressing the emotional havoc they wreak as well. CBD's anti-inflammatory and mood-balancing properties can be really supportive.

GETTING THE MUNCHIES: FACT OR FICTION?

The answer? A little bit of both. The concept of "the munchies" — the idea that using cannabis makes you want to snack — is all about THC-focused cannabis. THC can stimulate the appetite, along with its cousin cannabigerol (CBG), another important cannabinoid found in the plant.

Most of the appetite stimulation comes from the terpenes (certain plant chemicals) in that particular cannabis. Because cannabis contains terpenes in such high quantities, it has more of this reputation than almost any other plant medicine does. Full-spectrum CBD hemp flower, with the same terpene profile as THC cannabis, may have similar effects. Myrcene (found in mango, thyme, and citrus), beta-caryophyllene (found in pepper, hops, and basil) and limonene (found in citrus, juniper, and peppermint) can also be important in appetite stimulation.

However, the right terpene profile in both hemp and cannabis can have an appetite-suppressing effect. Humulene is one of the more common terpenes found in cannabis and hemp that has appetite-suppressing qualities. It's also found in hops and coriander.

Relieving Anorexia

Anorexia is characterized by the loss or lack of appetite for food. It's a medical condition and emotional disorder that appears as an obsessive desire to lose weight by refusing to consume food. It can often be coupled with *body dysmorphia*, where patients don't perceive that they've lost enough weight, even if their body mass index (BMI) is in the dangerously underweight category. CBD in one form or another may be able to address a wide variety of anorexia symptoms and common contributing factors.

Anorexia isn't really about food. Food is the control mechanism for dealing with emotional problems. People with anorexia often perceive being thin with a sense of self-worth. So the treatment really needs to center on both the emotional characteristics that lead people to control their food consumption and the behaviors associated with the condition, like excessive exercise and the misuse of diet aids, diuretics, enemas, and laxatives.

Gaining weight

Weight gain is an important piece for people with anorexia to regain their health. It's actually the first step to recovery. Too little weight on the body can weaken the immune system, create an overall fragility, and leave a person feeling perpetually fatigued. The terpenes (specific plant chemicals; see Chapter 2) in CBD combined with the terpenes in certain foods can stimulate the appetite. This double whammy is a beautiful opportunity to potentially help patients begin to gain weight. Generally, the process of refeeding begins with "the right" foods.

REMEMBER

Many of the factors of anorexia are actually behaviors of starvation. So although the emotional components may seem like the first fix, getting the body out of starvation mode is actually more important.

TIP

VeloBar CBD has little snack pack options and protein bars that contain CBD and are organic, vegan, gluten-free, soy-free, and non-GMO. Alternatively, CBD honey provides a multitude of beneficial nutrients and sugars to provide energy. Kitchen Toke is a cannabis-focused brand that makes really nice honey, where the bees that create the honey actually also pollinate the hemp plants that the CBD comes from. The brand Groovy Butter makes a variety of nut butters that are packed full of healthy plant-based proteins. Ojai Energetics makes its own CBD coconut oil, which is a great base for anything and can be added to beverages for a blast of healthy fat. It's the ultimate brain food and tastes great in a coffee, rich tea, or cacao beverage. These products are available on each brand's respective website.

Boosting appetite

As I note earlier in the chapter, some foods have the right terpene profiles to help stimulate appetite, and adding a dose of CBD to them can up the ante. The three main terpenes here are myrcene, beta-caryophyllene, and limonene. The strongest crossover of terpenes is myrcene and limonene because both occur in citrus. For the most part, the remaining terpene profiles you want come from herbs, including thyme, juniper, basil, peppermint, and black pepper. Even at a glance, you can probably see the yummy potential.

TIP

When I look at that list, I see the makings of a fabulous homemade salad dressing.

1. **Start with CBD olive oil.**

    Potli brand makes a great one, or use olive oil and add a dose of full-spectrum CBD oil. You can find instructions for infusing CBD oil in Chapter 4.

2. Zest and juice a lemon.

Add the fresh lemon juice to the oil in a one-to-one ratio to make the base. Add the lemon zest to taste.

3. Add salt and pepper.

I recommend pink Himalayan salt because it contains more calcium, potassium, magnesium, and iron than table salt. Even trace amounts are better than none. Be sure to use freshly cracked black pepper — the more, the better. (*Note:* The pre-cracked or granulated pepper doesn't have the same benefits because it's already oxidized and often has fillers.)

4. Add thyme and/or basil.

Give them a fine chop first.

Of course, you can add anything else that sounds good for taste — for example, a dash of honey for sweetness or a bit of Dijon mustard for spiciness and to mimic the flavor of a Caesar dressing. Any number of vinegars can provide a little bit more zest than just the aforementioned lemon. If you're going to use vinegar, I highly recommend an apple cider vinegar because that variety can be beneficial for digestive healing. You may find a bit more zest might require a little more oil, so taste as you go for balance. Lastly, if you're open to it, consider using an egg yolk in the base. This incredible protein boost can be a valuable asset when you're looking to gain weight. (Just do me a solid and make sure to wash the eggshell in warm water with antibacterial soap first.)

If you decide to go this route and don't want to use CBD olive oil, just make sure you're using a full-spectrum CBD tincture. Anything labeled to enhance mood is likely going to have the right terpene profile.

TIP

Now if that sounds like too much work, find a full-spectrum CBD supplement that can be consumed before mealtime to take the edge off and release level anxiety. If you can find one with a "mood-enhancing" profile, it will be a good extra boost.

LINKING CBD AND APPETITE

The results of studies on how CBD affects appetite run the gamut from "stimulating" to "suppressing." My experience and the view of some of the research I admire most suggest CBD can suppress appetite. This property is also presented in CBD's cannabinoid cousin THCV. (And no the "V" isn't a typo; I am not talking about THC. THCV is not psychoactive.) In future product evolution, we will see a combination of these two cannabinoids. The truth is that the outside factors are what CBD can stimulate and balance.

Regulating mealtime anxiety

Anxiety in people with anorexia often correlates to a fear of gaining weight. So at mealtime in particular, addressing the stress and anxiety of eating on a biological level however possible is important.

CBD can help physiologically. The volume of notable, experiential evidence around relieving anxiety, coupled with the right combination of appetite-stimulating terpenes (see the later section "Boosting appetite"), can lead to an opportunity to address two behaviors in one. For people with severe cases of anorexia, the perception of consuming anything orally is a challenge. The idea of the mouth as a vehicle for swallowing or eating can conjure up negative images and feelings, so any kind of CBD medicine in snack form, like snack foods, might be tough. Should that be the case, go with something inhalable, such as a vape or an inhaler. Another alternative is a transdermal patch. Any of these options could be the best way to relieve anxiety and support anti-inflammatory actions in the body.

If consuming food is an acceptable option, popular suggested snacks for transitioning into food, such as nut butters, are available with CBD in them. Otherwise, other CBD medicine taken orally, such as a tincture or a gel cap, may be a good go-to, especially before mealtime. In any case, there are many ways to get CBD into the system, and the best method is the one that the patient is willing to take.

Limiting the Psychological Effects of Bulimia

Though similar in many ways to anorexia (see the earlier section "Relieving Anorexia"), bulimia has its own special characteristics. It, too, is an emotional disorder with core issues of body image distortion and an obsessive desire to lose weight. *Bulimia* is characterized by excessive overeating followed by depression that leads to purging or fasting. The depressive aspects of bulimia are coupled with guilt and shame and also come with stress and anxiety. CBD may be able to alleviate all these issues in one way or another.

Dealing with the depression

The antidepressive qualities of CBD may make it an important component in treating bulimia — not just as a supplement but potentially also as an element in the food consumed by people with bulimia. In the early stages of managing bulimia, a supplemental form of CBD may be best to ensure the person gets enough

CBD into the bloodstream. If a person eats CBD in a snack and then purges shortly thereafter, the CBD likely won't have had time to get through the digestive system and into the blood. Likewise, if a person eats the CBD snack, and then binges on more food, the congestion in the digestives system of excesses of food will make it hard for the CBD in the snack to compete and get into the bloodstream in enough of a concentration before it is passed through and out of the system.

Mints, gums, and *sublinguals* (a form held under the tongue; see Chapter 7) may be the best starting point because they're quick acting and have the benefit of not looking, sounding, or feeling like a "food." Because of these factors, they might be best received. Favour Gum helps address the sublingual action of getting CBD into the bloodstream more quickly. Mints like Mr. Moxey's Relief mint with ginger are a great option here as well because the ginger is soothing to the digestive tract.

TIP

Dissolve the mints in your mouth slowly because this gives the dissolving CBD the best opportunity to come into contact with the blood vessels in the mouth and then get into the bloodstream.

A chocolate bar may be another good option. Really great quality raw cacao (dark chocolate) has mood-boosting properties, so combined with CBD in a CBD-infused cacao can be a real antidepressive.

TIP

I also tend to start my day with a cacao beverage for energy and a mood boost. I've included the recipe in Chapter 17.

Counteracting anxiety

The anti-anxiety aspects of CBD may be really beneficial in treating bulimia. Anxiety and depressive characteristics are chemically linked. That's why medications for anxiety and depression are often somewhat similar and/or prescribed together.

I note in the preceding section that gum is an opportunity to get CBD in the bloodstream more quickly. It's also a calming form that's easy to consume. People with anxiety sometimes exhibit fidgety-ness (a highly technical term) that may be well served by chewing gum. (Fun fact: Dating back to World War I, chewing gum was included in soldiers' rations as a way to calm nerves and manage stress.)

TIP

Favour Gum comes in a 10-milligram serving size. That's a great dose as a starting point and can be taken multiple times a day, quite easily, if needed.

Inducing sleep

People with bulimia may notice severely disrupted sleep patterns. Specifically, these folks often experience insomnia. Some people also do their bingeing when they wake up during disrupted sleep, so addressing opportunities for consistent sleep patterns is important. Interestingly enough, sleep deprivation from disrupted sleep patterns can affect not only the metabolism but also food regulation and response.

REMEMBER

Clinically, insomnia is related to an increased risk of eating disorders. Conversely, eating disorders are related to disrupted sleep patterns. Whether the chicken or the egg comes first here may not matter as much as figuring out how to improve sleep patterns. This piece is vital for ultimately getting the body's chemistry back on track and processing everything properly.

Some studies have indicated that getting a good night's rest can require as much as 300 to 600 milligrams of CBD. CBD can affect the release of cortisol, which is the body's stress response hormone. Levels of cortisol that are too high during rest periods can prevent sleep or create moments of sleeplessness.

However, I'd tend to say that 300 milligrams of CBD for anyone's body to achieve a state of rest and sleep may be overkill. I've seen some great results with CBD as a sleep aid for many of the people whom I've worked with. Multiple variables in the body create a level of sleeplessness in people with bulimia. Any treatment needs to be considerate toward those other biological factors. The best results in all walks of life, I believe, come from finding balance in diversity. So rather than taking one ingredient at really high doses, I much prefer taking multiple ingredients that complement one another together in moderate doses.

TIP

For this reason, I really like the sleep-focused brand Proper. It has a couple of different capsule forms that contain a variety of complementary medicines to achieve greater and deeper sleep. If capsules aren't for you, another brand called Winged CBD has a gel cap called Relief that has a formulation I can really get behind. It also has a CBD gummy that has really quality complementary ingredients. Both of these companies have their own websites with all the details on dosing, and my company Poplar (www.shop-poplar.com) carries them both as well.

Calming Nausea

Oh, nausea! The queasy feeling in your stomach that's sometimes a precursor to vomiting. In all senses, it's just so unpleasant. No one is immune to nausea, and no matter the cause, the remedies are likely always the same. Though no studies to date can point to CBD as a remedy for nausea, a long history of cannabis use for cancer patients looking for relief from chemotherapy can attest otherwise.

Mother's little helper: CBD and morning sickness

Speaking from experience, I can say that morning sickness is the farthest thing from what you want to feel while pregnant. So many other changes are going on in your body that are confusing enough as it is. Feeling nauseous is just icing on the cake.

The real problem here, though, is what can you take that will make you feel better and not compromise your baby? It's a real conundrum. Many Western medical practitioners suggest steering clear of natural medicines, so knowing what to do is hard. My nausea was limited, and I was already taking CBD for supplemental reasons, so seeking out a separate CBD treatment seemed to have little upside for me. That doesn't mean CBD can't be the right and the best thing for you if you're experiencing morning sickness. Like anything else, if you do go this route, go slow and low with your CBD and pair it with other ingredients that are supportive (such as ginger and honey).

TIP

Consider a CBD honey (or, alternately, manuka honey that you add full-spectrum CBD oil to) in a ginger tea served warm and sipped slowly. Rosebud or Lily both have high-concentration, full-spectrum hemp extracts in travel sizes so that you can test it out. My favorite brands of honey are Potli and Kitchen Toke. Another great option here is Mr. Moxey's Relief mints, which contain ginger. They're great to suck on and allow for slow sublingual absorption.

REMEMBER

The reality about CBD and pregnancy-related conditions is that research is in its infancy (great pun, I know!). In Chapter 14, I discuss using CBD during pregnancy. Jump ahead for a broader picture of use and considerations. I would also encourage you to find a doctor who practices in the space of natural medicines and alternative medicines and who has experience in addressing the challenging symptoms of being pregnant with natural treatments. For a bit more on finding a doctor, look at Chapter 5. Research, specifically as it relates to CBD and cannabis and pregnancy, is becoming more and more a topic of interest, so new data will likely be coming to light even by the time this book makes it to print. Keep your eyes peeled for new research.

Correcting chronic nausea

The history of cannabis as a treatment for chronic nausea goes back far longer in history than I'm sure you care to read at this point. But it appears in traditional Ayurvedic medicine texts dating back over 2,000 years. In the United States, just before the early days of California's statewide legalization in the 1990s, AIDS/HIV and cancer patients were using cannabis for relief from nausea, among other reasons. Believe it or not, that's actually how I got into this business. My mother was prescribed medical cannabis by my grandfather (a San Francisco pediatrician) to help her relieve nausea induced by chemotherapy. This was full-spectrum, THC-containing cannabis, smoked in all its glory.

In the early days, there were, of course, treats like brownies and such. However, when you're feeling a little nauseous, I don't know that brownies are the first thing on your radar. Inhaling CBD flower may provide the same benefits with a quicker onset. It may even keep you from vomiting. Head to Chapter 7 for more on the various inhalation forms.

TIP

If you suffer from chronic nausea and have access to a medical or adult-use dispensary, see whether you can find a full-spectrum cannabis flower or hemp flower with really high concentrations of CBD and really low concentrations of THC. (See Chapter 6 for more on both dispensaries and the legalities of THC.) I can't promise you that that's the ticket, but really low doses of THC and high doses of CBD to counteract the feelings of THC may be a viable solution. A mint, something that dissolves in your mouth, or a fast-acting, full-spectrum tincture may do the same thing here.

If you're looking for more creative solutions that go past plain flower, look for complementary medicines such as mint, lemon, and ginger. Plenty of value-added hemp and cannabis products have those three additives.

Reducing seasickness and motion sickness

Motion sickness and seasickness are a conflict between the senses — that is, your brain isn't making sense of the information your senses are providing. Your eyes are seeing things move in front of them, but they're also moving, and your muscles are coordinating your body to shift with the movements of whatever is carrying you. The sounds are changing, and I could just get sick *thinking* about all of that.

Lots of things can be triggers, such as rides in cars, boats, airplanes, and amusement park rides. Initial queasiness can lead to dizziness and nausea and then vomiting.

CBD's interaction with serotonin can potentially help relieve the body's response to nausea associated with motion sickness. Combine that with a perception that CBD can help with balance, and some brands are claiming that CBD can provide relief.

TIP

The fastest-acting method of CBD delivery, smoking, is likely a no-go in most scenarios that bring on motion sickness. A mint or a chewable gum, such as the ones I recommend throughout this chapter, is a good option here as well. Because attacks of motion sickness and seasickness tend to happen on the go, make sure you have your remedy stashed on you when you may be getting into situations that can induce nausea. You may even want to leave a stash in your car so you always have it. If you're almost certain you'll experience some sort of motion sickness, take a dose of CBD well before you hop in the car or on the plane, just to make sure that it's already had time to activate in your system. That may be as much as two hours depending on the delivery method (see Chapter 7).

Chapter 12

Coping with Muscular and Physical Ailments

CBD is a powerful and world-renowned pain reliever. One of its most studied and celebrated functions is how it quells inflammation. CBD's anti-inflammatory properties address topical and internal concerns. In preliminary studies, CBD has been linked to expedited cell turnover, which means it's an ideal treatment for inflammatory concerns that proliferate quickly across the skin and in cells.

In this chapter, I explore the effects of CBD on muscle recovery. I also discuss how CBD can relieve fibromyalgia, asthmatic symptoms, migraines, and diabetes and insulin resistance. Solutions range from topical to ingestible.

Connecting CBD and Muscle Recovery

Reducing muscle inflammation and increasing blood flow are critical for muscle recovery, and CBD has been indicated as being able to do both. No wonder the marketplace is full of CBD sport balms, tinctures, and related products.

Utilizing hemp-derived dermal solutions

The topical solutions for localized relief are abundant. You can easily find special-ized lotions, sprays, balms, salves, and even transdermal patches that particularly target your specific ailments.

TIP

I tend to be a fan of topicals that allow you to massage them into the body. The rubbing and kneading allow for an extra circulation, which sends oxygen to your muscles and in turn boosts recovery. My company Poplar (www.shop-poplar.com) offers a great selection of muscle recovery solutions, one of them being Thera-One's Recover. It's a great CBD lotion with complementary ingredients from arnica to clove bud oil and more.

When you're on the go, transdermal patches can offer similar, albeit slightly dif-ferent, relief.

Soothing post-workout soreness internally

The solutions in the preceding section are great for general post-workout sore-ness or muscle exertion, too. Simply take a shower post-workout and apply one right after. But for whole body relief, an internal remedy is best.

Some people prefer to take CBD *before* athletic endeavors, depending on the form and the dose, because they know it'll kick in sometime within the workout and have residual effects. Others prefer to take an internal remedy after their work-outs, knowing that the benefits will kick in as their bodies are beginning to recover.

If you're still on the fence, I recommend dipping your toe into post-workout CBD remedies slowly. They're a great way to get ahead of soreness and potentially reduce stiffness and discomfort.

Pampering overworked joints with bath bombs or muscle soaks

You can take the fast, easy route and slather on a balm or salve. Or you can hop aboard the self-care train and really luxuriate in your CBD experience. A whole host of CBD bath bombs and muscle soaks (similar to bath salts) can really take muscle trauma recovery to the next level.

A good bath bomb contains a volume of CBD appropriate for muscle recovery and overworked joints. They also generally have sodium bicarbonate (baking soda) and a bit of magnesium, typically in the form of Epsom salt. To entice your nose, companies often include essential oils or flower-derived fragrances as well. These botanical additives certainly do add an aromatherapy component that can be relaxing.

The CBD volume you're looking for varies based on the experience you're after:

>> **Subtle relaxation:** 50 milligrams

>> **Muscle relaxation:** 75 milligrams

>> **Spa-style recovery soak:** Between 150 and 200 milligrams

The mineral ingredients are the most important additions to CBD products for maximum effectiveness. Magnesium is essential because it has been proven through generations to increase muscle recovery. Your product needs to have one to two cups of Epsom salt to achieve the magnesium benefits required for full-body recovery. Some soaks even contain additional forms of salt to add to the mineral benefits. Sodium bicarbonate absorbs all the toxins your system is releasing into the water so you don't reabsorb them as you soak. And that's helpful, because you'll be soaking for more than 20 minutes to achieve the full benefits of the bath.

TIP

If you find yourself with a soak that doesn't have enough Epsom salt, just add an extra cup. You can buy Epsom salt at your local drugstore.

TIP

So many great soaks are out on the market. I'm partial to the Verte Essentials spa-style soaks because they have all the ingredients in the right volume for full-body recovery. They're on the fancier side, though, so something a little more accessible to use on a regular basis is a Vertly brand or Empower Bodycare brand product. These have a great volume of beneficial ingredients and good value. All are available at my company Poplar (www.shop-poplar.com). Papa & Barkley brand has a great soak as well. Just add a little extra Epsom and about a tablespoon of baking soda for maximum benefits.

Note: You can find a few other CBD topicals, generally in spray format, that contain a concentration of magnesium. Vertly brand has a nice option. Though they may address a topical and regional level of pain, relief doesn't seep down as deep as you want. Sprays aren't likely to get down to the root issue and address it systematically as a bath soak may. So magnesium sprays are a great quick fix on the go, but to go deeper and to really pamper yourself, grab a magnesium-rich, mineral-fortified CBD bath soak. It takes recovery and relaxation to the next level.

Relaxing the Symptoms of Fibromyalgia

Fibromyalgia is a bone and muscle condition with a lot of symptoms:

» Widespread pain and localized tenderness

» Chronic touch sensitivity

» Sleeplessness/fatigue

» Mood issues

» Brain fog

Fibromyalgia is often triggered by psychological or physical stressors. The silver lining is that CBD is the gift that keeps on giving for fibromyalgia patients. Dosing here is going to be scaled relative to the severity of symptoms that any patient may be addressing. Many of the these symptoms are discussed in more depth in other chapters, so I will refrain from being redundant and instead lead you to other sections and chapters.

Resting easier

The good news is that CBD can alleviate the sleeplessness associated with fibromyalgia. It helps the body relax into a deeper sleep. Better sleep means reduced anxiety, tension, and restlessness. Getting better rest and deeper sleep ultimately helps address some of the fatigue concerns that also affect those with fibromyalgia.

TIP

You can find further details on sleeplessness in Chapter 11 in the section on bulimia, and again in Chapter 13 surrounding mood disorders and PTSD. (Chapter 13 also covers mood disorders in general.)

Alleviating pain (without getting hooked)

The reason CBD is so great for fibromyalgia is that it helps address the inflammation that leads to the trademark acute pain. Because fibromyalgia is a chronic condition, a solution that doesn't create dependency is a top priority.

One of the beautiful realities of CBD is that it isn't habit forming. Unlike other medicines, it doesn't necessarily build up in the system and create increased tolerance over time. In fact, when you find the dose that's right for you, your body will likely cement it as your dosage amount for the foreseeable future. So far, research has indicated that the only risk of dependency is the desire to continue to use it for relief from your condition.

CONSIDERING TRANSDERMAL PATCHES FOR FIBROMYALGIA

You can address pain on your terms by selecting the solution that's most tailored to your needs. Another way of getting CBD into the bloodstream (besides a topical cream or balm) is a transdermal patch applied to the affected region. Transdermal patches offer quick uptake into the bloodstream. For some, they may be the preferred method to treat the widest discomfort and fibromyalgia as a whole. Finding the proper dose is key.

Clearing brain fog

Case studies have indicated that CBD can benefit chronic patients looking to treat "fibro fog." CBD's many functions include nourishing and protecting the brain. Increasing blood flow and oxygenation to the brain helps with clarity, and this result may be achieved with CBD use because a decrease of inflammation can lead to cleared pathways for blood and oxygen transport. Because the brain is what's at play here and it has historically been linked to the gut, ingestible remedies are the best bet in addressing this condition or related side effects.

Activating Asthma Relief

Asthma is a chronic condition that affects patients young and old. It causes the airways into the lungs to narrow because of an increase in inflammation. All things considered from previous chapters, as we have explored CBD as a tool for inflammation relief, it seems only fitting that we explore CBD as a remedy.

Looking at the lungs

Studies have indicated that CBD may be a possible *bronchodilator,* which causes the air passages in the lungs to widen. Ultimately, research has indicated that CBD in conjunction with two other cannabinoids (delta 8-THC and delta 9-THC) most effectively support bronchodilation. Asthma attacks come on quickly and therefore require quick relief. Taken in the proper form (in this case, some form of inhalation), CBD may relax the constricted lung muscles while helping decrease the inflammation. Ultimately, this action potentially can unblock constricted airways. The best potential combination for asthma flare-ups will be a combination inhaler of THC and CBD, which will only be available through a regulated retail destination. Brands available will vary by state. Not enough research exists to indicate whether or not CBD itself will be a viable preventative and maintenance tool for asthma. Since the airway constriction can be in part due to inflammation, it is possible that CBD used as a supplement on a regular basis may prevent more frequent flare-ups. However, there's currently no hard to suggest that is the case.

Breathing better

CBD has been recognized as an anti-spasmatic. And because one of the unfortunate side effects of asthma is *bronchospasms* (where the muscles lining the airways tighten), the asthma community is researching CBD more and more. CBD's anti-inflammatory properties can potentially provide more lasting relief from the muscle spasms associated with asthma.

REMEMBER

Timing plays a factor. It's really about finding the right form and being able to access it at the right time. Delivery methods with longer onset times aren't likely to help unless you know you'll be in a situation that may trigger your asthma and can plan ahead accordingly. A better option may be an inhaler. Omura devices offer a smokeless combustion of flower, which could be better than a traditional smoking apparatus that puts smoke into your lungs. You can read more about the various CBD delivery methods and their onset times in Chapter 7.

Increased relief from inflammation throughout the lungs and improved delivery of oxygen to the lungs (because of increased blood flow) are all benefits of CBD. These positive effects help with breathing better and more deeply. Rapid inflammation can be another contributor to an asthmatic flare-up. And in these instances, a doctor is likely to prescribe an anti-inflammatory that's intended to decongest airways over a duration. CBD may evolve to be one of these anti-inflammatory treatments.

TIP

CBD aside, small changes in your habits can have large and helpful ripple effects. Studies show that taking deep, intentional breaths more often increases clarity, energy, and your overall quality of life.

A few CBD inhalers are on the market, but many of them are from medically unregulated vendors. Do yourself a huge favor and emphatically research. Less traditional forms of inhalers include sniffers for the nose, which contain essential oils, or a simple inhalation of vapors via a vaporizer. And when I say *vaporizer* in this particular sense, I don't mean a vape that looks like a cigarette or a pen. I'm talking about a vaporizer that forms and vaporizes the substance for inhalation but, unlike the popular "vape" that dominates the public eye, does not require a carrier agent or other natural or synthetic additives. It simply vaporizes the cannabis or hemp flower.

TIP

Make & Mary brand has a beautiful line of inhalers for sniffing the essential oils and extracts from not only hemp CBD but also complementary plants. They are actually one of our better-selling products on my company's website, www.shop-poplar.com.

Mitigating Migraines and Other Headaches

Migraines are more than just a headache; they can be debilitating on a variety of levels. Unfortunately, I'm speaking from personal experience. They contribute to anxiety, sleeplessness, lack of focus, fatigue, and more. Early clinical surveys have suggested that CBD is helping migraine sufferers in a really significant way by reducing the frequency and onset of their headaches. For some, it potentially prevents further worsening after a migraine has already begun. Like in all other areas of CBD research, more information is necessary. But as with any difficult-to-treat condition, any relief at all is still relief.

Menstrual migraines

Menstrual migraines are a touch different in that they're said to be a result of a dip in estrogen and progesterone around the start of the menstrual cycle. They come with throbbing pain, nausea, and sometimes other symptoms. Because they're much more predictable than migraines that just come on at any time or have outside triggers, you can anticipate and plan ahead. Prepare for this time of the month with a regular supplemental dose of CBD, in whatever form — ingesting enough CBD to get ahead of it is the ticket.

Make sure the bioavailability of the form you're consuming is significant enough. For that, you need to know your dose not just for supplementation but also for achieving deeper relief. If you know your supplemental dose is 10 milligrams (a standard base to build off of), double it and take 20 milligrams two or three times a day. If you change forms here, be sure to accommodate bioavailability changes. For example, a 10-milligram supplement in tincture form is like a 30-millgram gel cap. It just takes a little math. Refer to Chapter 8 for more details on bioavailability if you want to make sure you're achieving the proper dose.

Quelling stress-induced headaches

CBD use may mitigate stress-induced headaches and migraines. One of the more widely accepted benefits of CBD is stress relief. With overwhelming anecdotal evidence, CBD has largely been adopted as a potential anxiety soother as well.

Finding a ritual or a routine for taking internal doses of CBD may help keep the stress that triggers these headaches (and thus the headaches themselves) at bay.

To treat stress-induced headaches after they've started, find a form of CBD that offers quick action. Your options include the smoking, inhaling, vaping, or sublingual categories (see Chapter 7). Stay away from CBD edibles if you've already started to experience the onset of the pain; they take too long to kick in. (That said, if you've already taken your quick-onset CBD solution and know that a CBD cookie will make you feel better psychologically, go for it.)

Upgrading from traditional prescription treatments

WARNING

Have a conversation with your medical practitioner before making any changes to your prescription treatments.

An incredible amount of preliminary research looks to identify CBD as an alternative to what you may already be working with. Any sort of prescription treatment that you've been relying on for quite some time may have a dependency factor. The myriad side effects associated with many pharmaceuticals can be detrimental throughout a lifetime. Getting rid of nasty and unwanted side effects may even require additional medication. It's a vicious cycle.

If tweaking your prescriptions and supplements isn't a matter of life and death (and for some people it is), exploring what's already present in the CBD market as a solution for your particular condition may be an incredible opportunity for you.

Dealing with Diabetes and Insulin Resistance

Ultimately *diabetes* is a chronic condition that affects how your body turns food into energy. Food is broken down into a form of sugar that accesses the bloodstream to provide energy. There are two types of diabetes: Type 1 diabetics don't produce insulin, and type 2 diabetics don't respond to insulin. *Insulin resistance*, a characteristic of type 2 diabetes, can also be present without the actual presentation of diabetes. It can be genetic and environmental. Remission is possible (a cure, not so much, at least not yet).

Examining insulin resistance and CBD

More technically, type 1 diabetes is a compromise in insulin production, which happens in the pancreas. The body turns most foods into glucose that then requires transport from the bloodstream to the cells for energy. The hormone *insulin* is that transport. *Insulin resistance* occurs when the cells in your body don't respond well to insulin and it builds up elsewhere.

Preliminary research has indicated that CBD shows promise in reducing insulin resistance, which is directly in relation to type 2 diabetes. The body's endocannabinoid system (see Chapter 3) is said to play a role in how you respond to insulin by either increasing or decreasing sensitivity. Given that some people with diabetes take insulin, whether CBD is helpful or unhelpful is hard to say. It may be responsible for peaks and valleys, which are ultimately what people with diabetes are trying to avoid. Research related to CBD and other cannabinoids is promising, but it's still too early to tell.

Ask your doctor about trying CBD for managing insulin resistance for type 2 diabetes. Avoid any of those nasty additives like sugars and flavorings. Staying away from the snacks, treats, and edibles altogether may be your best bet.

Preventing diabetes with CBD

Studies done on obese diabetic mice found that those treated with CBD had a lower risk of developing diabetes. But humans aren't mice. As I note in the preceding section, no serious studies to date have indicated that CBD helps prevent diabetes. However, some anecdotal references have pointed to potential prevention as well as the treatment of inflammation and pain associated with diabetes.

Regulating blood sugar levels through appetite suppression

The biggest concern around diabetes is regulating blood sugar (officially, *blood glucose*) levels. To date, no significant studies have indicated that CBD controls blood sugar. Those in a prediabetic state who have trouble regulating sugar intake may be able to curb cravings by taking the proper form of CBD and complementing ingredients as an appetite suppressant.

REMEMBER

This is worth saying again: CBD itself does not regulate blood sugar levels. It's more of a tool to help you regulate consumption habits that may spike blood sugar levels.

IN THIS CHAPTER

» **Exploring the differences between anxiety and stress**

» **Diving into how CBD can treat the effects of depression**

» **Perusing CBD's effects on the symptoms of post-traumatic stress disorder**

» **Treating aspects of addictions**

» **Breaking down CBD's potential for treating bipolar disorder**

Chapter **13**

Helping with Emotional, Mood, and Mental Disorders

Many emotional, mood, and mental disorders can be quite hard to treat. Prescription drugs on the market often offer short-term solutions over long-term durations. However, merely providing stability isn't enough. The ultimate goal in addressing these kinds of conditions and disorders is to work through and get over them instead of suppressing or keeping them at bay.

Improving mood disorders often involves lengthy and sometimes lifelong steps. Many theories suggest that treating these types of disorders requires a variety of therapeutic approaches. For example, within the Western tradition, "successful psychiatric treatment" usually includes a psychotherapist by default. When these integrative therapies aren't necessarily an option, exploring other potential remedies on the market that may go beyond the traditional suppress-and-carry-on mentality seems fitting.

In this chapter, I look at the potential for CBD remedies for depression, anxiety, general mood challenges, PTSD, addiction therapies, and bipolar disorder.

REMEMBER

Although no company is going to specifically come out and say that it offers relief from depression, or any condition, in a roundabout way it'll find an opportunity to suggest that may be a possibility. The FDA ultimately regulates the space and has a say on the kinds of claims that companies in the natural product space can make. CBD companies can't say that they "do" anything.

Ultimately, find a form of CBD to consume that brings you joy. Because if you're looking to take something to encourage a better mood in your life, don't you think the experience of consuming it should also inspire positive feelings? You can read more about delivery forms in Chapter 7.

Identifying the Differences between Stress and Anxiety

Stress and anxiety are often coupled together because they have many similar symptoms. That said, they are very different and require a different style of treatment. I break them both down for you here so that you can see clearly how they are different, and then I discuss the treatment benefits for both CBD and anxiety as well as CBD and stress.

Stress, while it might manifest in symptoms similar to anxiety, is actually not the same at all. Anxiety can be a lifelong condition that requires constant care and upkeep. Neither stress nor anxiety are technically mood disorders, but since symptoms can manifest similarly to mood disorders, I felt this chapter was the best place to address the conditions. Likewise, anxiety and other mood disorders like depression can be treated similarly with pharmaceutical medications. Determining if you are truly experiencing stress or anxiety is crucial to setting out on the correct treatment plan.

Processing stress so that it doesn't lead to anxiety

Stress presents with a series of symptoms, including fatigue, anger and irritability, sleeplessness, and more. Unlike anxiety, there is a trigger, a stressor event or events. When that trigger is alleviated, the feeling of stress subsides. Persistent stressors can lead to anxiety if they go unmitigated, so it is important to take stress as the warning sign that it is and address it.

Stress is your body's way of telling you, *"Look out! You have gone too far."* If you don't heed these warning signs, your body goes into overdrive, flooding your system with the neuro signals that you should continue to be in this state of overdrive. Pay attention to these signs and slow down. By eliminating or mitigating the stressor, or working to find ways through the experience, you run a better chance of not wreaking havoc on the rest of your body. Additional tools such as exercise, sleep, and reasonable work hours can be helpful.

Taking natural medicine like CBD and a host of other plants containing chemicals to relax the body can be helpful. Of these chemicals specifically, I have discussed terpenes already, so refer to Chapter 2 to better understand what to look for in ingredient combinations. Additional complementary plant medicines, referred to as *nervines,* which support the nervous system, help de-stress the system and will make great ingredient additions to CBD products. All nervines are helpful for reducing the effects of stress and the symptoms on your system. These plants include chamomile, kava, valerian, catnip, lemon balm, lavender and more.

TIP

Barbari brand makes a nice smoke blend that has a combination of stress-relieving plants. It can be consumed as a joint or with the smokeless Omura device. Verte Essentials, the brand I formulated and own, also has a nice tincture called Focus, which is great for mild stress and clarity because of its CBD and host of other stress-relieving botanicals. It's exclusively sold on shop-poplar.com.

Unpacking the causes and treatments around anxiety

To be specific, anxiety is characterized as a condition of chronic worry that interferes with one's functionality. Anxiety disorders vary in degree from mild symptoms persisting beyond a six-month period to severe worry and fear, preventing someone from partaking in everyday activities. *Generalized anxiety disorder* (GAD), *social anxiety disorder* (SAD), and *post-traumatic stress disorder* (PTSD), covered later in the chapter, are all forms of anxiety. In these varying levels of anxiety, patients may experience the following:

>> Heart palpitations

>> Tension

>> Excessive sweating

>> Irritability

>> Distorted thinking

>> Constant worry

- » Nervousness
- » Severe fear sensations
- » Irritability
- » Panic attacks

Anxiety, over the long term, affects your neurotransmitters. This interaction affects mood, appetite, digestion, and sleep patterns and can contribute to depressive behavior. Regular supplementation with CBD would interact with serotonin receptors and in turn boost mood. CBD has also been shown to decrease anxiety symptoms in patients in both high and low doses. Actual studies have been done in this area of scientific research, both on rats and on human patients. Success was acknowledged in the rats by monitoring a decrease in elevated heart rate. In human patients, a double-blind test with 400 milligrams of CBD against a placebo and patients receiving the CBD noted a decrease in anxiety symptoms.

You may note that this is a particularly large dose of CBD, relative to what else you might have read or the recommended dose on the back of most CBD product packages. I would tend to agree with you, but complex and severe symptoms can require considerable volume. This is not always the case, which is why I would still recommend you start low and go slow to find the appropriate dose.

Should you need a high dose, make sure you are choosing a form factor with high bioavailability to make sure you are maximizing your medicine for the volume you will require. This would mean an inhalable, smokable, or a tincture in form. For situations of quick onset, it's best to have something that's fast-acting as well, and any of the three are going to be the fastest to act.

Lily brand makes a great high-powered tincture with a 50-milligram serving. This could be a great starting point. Given that 50 milligrams can be quite high for some folks, I would recommend starting with a half dose in the evening to see if it makes you a bit drowsy. If you don't find yourself getting a little sleepy, go ahead and try that same dose during the day. You may find that you need to go with a full dose or even more for relief. Take note of the previous section where I outline some terpene combinations for stress relief, as they will have a similar effect on anxiety.

WARNING

While low doses of THC in your CBD may help with anxiety, generally speaking, high doses of THC may increase anxiety. Make sure you know the contents of the product you are consuming.

Exploring the effects (and side effects) of traditional anti-anxiety medication

Anxiety and depression are quite similar in that they both often coexist, and they both share a link to the brain's neurotransmitters, serotonin, and dopamine. Thus, both depression and anxiety are traditionally treated with the same types of medications. Due to the similarities and the crossover in treatment details, head to the next section for more info on the effects and side effects of traditional anti-depressants. Many studies cite CBD as having and exhibiting antidepressant-like characteristics.

Easing Depression

Many studies cite CBD as having and exhibiting antidepressant-like characteristics as well as anti-anxiety properties. Most of this evidence is a byproduct of findings from other studies around CBD and its therapeutic effects, but enough has been uncovered to encourage further exploration related to depression.

Examining the effects (and side effects) of traditional antidepressants

Traditional antidepressants are designed to balance the neurotransmitters in your brain (see the following section) to improve mood, sleep, appetite, and concentration. The drugs work temporarily while they're in your system but have no sustained effect after they've worn off, so they carry a risk of dependency and absolutely no guarantee or even likelihood of a cure.

Dependency isn't the only possible side effect. Other common complaints include

>> Sleeplessness, drowsiness, and fatigue

>> Mood swings

>> Dry mouth

>> *Brain zaps* (annoying but ultimately unharmful electrical sensations in the brain)

>> Sexual dysfunction

The later section "Combating the sexual side effects of mood modulating medications" has more on that last one, as well as info on how CBD may be able to counteract it.

This isn't to say that antidepressants (selective serotonin reuptake inhibitors, or SSRIs) don't have their place and aren't necessary or incredibly beneficial for some. I'm just emphasizing that new opportunities *are* on the horizon, as the following sections illustrate.

Helping your brain better respond to mood modulating systems in the body

Serotonin is the hormone responsible for feelings of happiness and well-being. It's known to stabilize mood and emotions. CBD can't increase serotonin levels per se, but it may affect how the receptors in your brain respond to existing serotonin levels. It's a "when life gives you lemons, make lemonade" sort of situation.

CBD also interacts with two other vital neurotransmitters, dopamine and glutamate. These two are responsible for the whole of your mood; between them, they regulate motivation, reward-seeking behaviors, and general cognition.

The combination of these three internal modulators is essential in identifying real potential antidepressant effects. The sheer stimulation effect of CBD, combined with an improved response system for the existing chemicals in the body, is exciting.

Modulating low moods and anxiety

CBD has been shown to have mood-modulating effects without the challenging side effects of traditional pharmaceutical drugs (see the earlier section "Examining the effects [and side effects] of traditional antidepressants"). The preliminary studies around CBD suggest that it can act as an antidepressant. Regular supplementation with CBD would interact with serotonin receptors and in turn boost mood. Keeping things regular, if you will, is a good thing for people who can swing from high to low on the mood spectrum. And indeed, a plethora of CBD products are marketed for that purpose alone.

I also suggest you find complementary ingredients to support antidepressive properties in the body. As I indicate in Chapter 10, linalool and limonene are both *terpenes* (plant chemicals) with anti-depressive benefits.

Verte's Pour le Sport line has a great limonene- and linalool-rich, full-spectrum CBD oil that can be used as a daily supplement. It's exclusively sold on shop-poplar.com, my company's website.

POSTPARTUM DEPRESSION

Postpartum depression (PPD), sometimes called the "baby blues," can be caused by a physical spike in hormones during pregnancy and a sharp drop-off of hormones post-delivery. Social and psychological changes as well can contribute to postpartum depression. This is not only a condition of the childbearing mother; dads and partners have been known to get it as well. PPD is often treated with antidepressants and/or anti-anxiety medication and counseling. You can find out more about pregnancy and CBD in Chapter 14.

Combating the sexual side effects of mood modulating medications

Antidepressants' side effects on the libido can range from loss of sexual desire to more physical manifestations like a lack of orgasm or erectile dysfunction. (So even the upside of not being depressed still may not be as fun.)

CBD's benefits can potentially help counteract the negative side effects of commonly prescribed pharmaceuticals, such as drowsiness, fatigue, and insomnia — all of which can turn you off and result in a decreased libido. It's still too early to tell for sure, but I say give it a whirl. What's the worst that can happen? It may help!

Calming the Symptoms of Post-Traumatic Stress Disorder

Post-traumatic stress disorder (PTSD) is a psychiatric disorder that manifests in people who have experienced tremendous trauma in their lives, such as witnessing a natural disaster or experiencing an act of war, other life-threatening situations, sexual violence, rape, or personal injury. PTSD is incredibly relative from individual to individual. The compounded stress in these individuals has far-reaching physiological implications as well as psychological manifestations. For the disorder to be addressed, the brain must be rewired or reset and both the mental and physical aspects improved. As a supportive step in recovery, CBD can lend a helping hand for many of the side effects of this condition.

Relieving the stress of painful memories

The painful memories associated with PTSD never go away. Even when they're no longer part of the conscious memory cycle, they still exist in the body's subconscious and physiological recollections. Humans have a very complex memory structure that extends far beyond the conscious brain.

But if CBD can help remediate the feelings of stress and anxiety associated with whatever caused the PTSD, that's a really important step forward.

TIP

I'd say that, from a supplemental standpoint, doses may need to be on the stronger side with a complementary dose of mood-boosting terpenes and ingredients to address these memories. I suggest a good, solid dose of extra strength, full-spectrum tincture, or whatever form makes you happiest. Double down and back it up with a dose of cacao drinkables (such as the ones in Chapter 17) to balance the adrenals and boost the production of *anandamide* (a cannabinoid native to the human body and also found in cacao). The pairing is a little blast of happiness.

Sweeping away stress and worry from nightmares

Some theories suggest the nightmares and unpleasant dreams associated with PTSD are the subconscious brain living a present-tense tale that induces fear, anxiety, and stress. Interruptions to a solid sleep state compromise the importance of working through a dream cycle. CBD has been reported time and time again to help with sleeplessness and insomnia. Ultimately, relaxing the body and the brain and alleviating stress and anxiety is paramount. Allowing the body an opportunity to release into a state of sleep is useful for many reasons. Melatonin and herbs that support the nervous system, like chamomile and lemon balm, can help work with the body and CBD to achieve a greater level of sleep.

Another complementary compound that can help sleep is THC. Even a really low ratio of THC to CBD, like 1:20, can really help the neurological components of achieving deep sleep. Because of national laws regarding THC, this kind of tincture is going to require you to have access to a medical or adult-use dispensary. But if the challenges are significant enough, seeking out that retail option is worth it. You can read more about both THC laws and dispensaries in Chapter 6.

TIP

Juna brand's Nightcap is a great option with full-spectrum benefits. It contains added relaxing ingredients like chamomile. The brand Mineral has a great product for sleep as well. A little bit goes a long way. Take the recommended dose for three nights and see how it treats you.

Another, non-CBD tip for promoting sleep: Avoid having any sugars right before bed (even up to a couple of hours before). This includes alcohol because it's likely to boost your blood sugar, spike your adrenals, and wake you up in the middle of the night. If you're inclined to have a bit of sugar or a glass of wine before bed anyway, consider eating a small handful of nuts to provide your body a little protein. The protein helps counteract that impending sugar spike.

Abolishing anger and irritability

Anger and irritability are a symptom of PTSD. Psychology says that experiencing trauma creates a feeling of violation that can leave patients feeling like they're out of control. PTSD also frequently leads to neurophysiological changes in the brain. The emotional processing center of the brain also modulates the fear response. This brain center can be overly reactive in PTSD patients.

The general calming effects of CBD can potentially help modulate a sense of anger and overwhelm. I'd say if anything, CBD provides the calm to take a deep breath and process this response for what it is. Let it pass, and carry on.

Addressing the Physical and Emotional Components of Addiction

Dependency has both psychological and physiological components. Physical or emotional stress and anxiety can trigger cycles of use for those with addictions. Habit-forming drugs that provide relief from physical or emotional stressors also perpetuate addiction. It can also be a side effect of chronic pain. Inevitably, it's all interlinked.

For some, this topic may be a bit controversial because CBD is associated with a regulated drug and was formerly regulated itself. CBD, however, isn't habit forming, and it also doesn't build up in the body and create a tolerance. Rather, after you find a dose to mediate a particular symptom or condition, that's where the dose stays. It's a beautiful thing.

Professionals have long considered addiction a disease. Alleviating the physical components of addiction doesn't necessarily get rid of the addiction itself. The potential for triggers, cravings, and relapse are always there.

Different addictions require different considerations. Alcohol isn't the same as opioids, which aren't the same as heroin, and so on.

CBD doesn't create a dependency and can help with anxiety and depression, which are two experiences that serve as contributors or triggers for relapse. If CBD can offer assistance in the physical and emotional space here, it seems like a good opportunity to try something that likely won't lead down the path to potential relapse.

Curbing heroin cravings

A 2019 study by the Recovery Research Institute tested CBD against a placebo with individuals suffering from heroin use disorder. The study indicated that those who received a dose of CBD had

>> Reduced cravings for heroin

>> A reduced level of anxiety for up to a week after

This is the only clinical trial to date with proper measures and the right protocol. As the marketplace opportunities continue to increase for CBD and the pharmaceutical companies get on board, you're likely to see more tests with similar structures looking to duplicate the results.

Treating opioid addiction

REMEMBER

The opioid epidemic is a crisis. Pharmaceutical drugs for pain relief create dependency. In turn, that dependency can lead to addiction and all else that follows in its wake. The best treatment here is prevention.

Social scientist (and dear friend of mine) Amanda Reiman, PhD, is responsible for some of the most incredible research around cannabis as an alternative to opioids. The bottom line is that full-spectrum cannabis with all the cannabinoids present, including THC and CBD, can provide incredible remediation from chronic pain without dependency. If you find yourself with an extra minute and a serious interest, look up her work online for more. Chapter 6 has details on the legalities of THC.

Reducing dependence on alcohol

Preliminary research indicates that using CBD in combination with alcohol use may reduce alcohol consumption. Additionally, CBD may reduce alcohol's negative effects on the body. All the studies to date have been done on mice, and clinical research is still needed, but much of the other research in regards to cannabis is in the same boat.

Alcoholism taxes the liver, causing inflammation there and in the brain. Because CBD seems to reduce oxidative stress and decrease inflammation (see Chapter 9), it may have similar effects on the oxidative stress and inflammation drinking causes on those organs.

TIP

I don't want to diminish alcoholism. I've been around it intimately. But I like alcohol for relaxation — as my unwind ritual at the end of the day — and I can often have more than one drink. Having been in the cannabis industry long enough to understand the benefits, though, I've evolved my ritual. Now one of my favorite ways to make a cocktail is with a little dose of CBD and sometimes a touch of THC. It provides me just the level of relaxation I want to calm down my day and keep me from anxiously fixating on checklists and to-do lists. It also keeps me from having another drink. I don't feel compelled to "keep" unwinding after one when I have the right combination of cannabis.

Many of my peers would far prefer an edible, a full-spectrum cannabis chocolate bar, or a puff off a joint or smokable device over alcohol almost any day. I have to say that those leaning in that direction are far more functional the following day than they would be if alcohol was their selected method for relaxation.

Assisting with Bipolar Disorder

Bipolar disorder (formerly called *manic depression*) is quite different from the mood disorders I describe earlier in the chapter, but it does have many similar symptoms: pain, sleeplessness, anxiety, and depressive characteristics. Other effects of the disorder include excessive mood swings, from super high highs to super low lows. CBD has antidepressant and anti-anxiety effects. It's also a pain and sleep aid and is shown to be promising for so many of these symptoms.

Remedying mood swings

Traditionally, a combination of mood-stabilizing medications, such as lithium, anticonvulsants, antipsychotics, and SSRIs, and lifelong therapy are in order to treat bipolar disorder. But intense mood stabilizers like lithium are often associated with an experience of numbness.

Adding CBD to this combination or cocktail of medications may or may not help from a processing standpoint. Like with other conditions where multiple medications are present, go through qualified medical practitioners to make decisions about what's best for you and what contraindications may be. The liver is responsible for processing so many medications; the last thing you want to do is overwork that beauty. Additional side effects can occur from taking medications that aren't complementary to one another.

REMEMBER

Everything I'm saying here is merely speculation on what may be possible with the further development of CBD as a potential mood modulator. If it seems like a good fit after you consider these points, regular supplementation with CBD starting slow and low is step one. Chapter 5 has details on supplementing.

Managing mania

The early stages of research around CBD as a whole have given incredible indications that CBD may interact with serotonin modulation. As I explain earlier in the chapter, serotonin is a neurotransmitter in the brain responsible, largely, for mood. Studies suggest that CBD interacts with your serotonin receptors, potentially prolonging the serotonin you do have in your system long enough to enjoy it a little bit more.

Disruptions in dopamine circuits, like the aforementioned serotonin circuitry, also appear to be connected to mental disorders of this nature. Both dopamine and serotonin receptors interact with CBD. Conversely, SSRIs and some other antidepressants responsible for blocking serotonin reuptake have been reported to induce manic episodes. So, this is a tricky space.

Using CBD as an adjunctive treatment

Lots of side effects to bipolar disorder are worth exploring for treatment. The myriad medications prescribed (in perpetuity) for this disorder come with their own side effects as well.

Inevitably, a whole host of synthetic medications promote wear and tear on the immune system. Inflammation is an immune system response, so exploring systematic inflammation relief seems prudent. Adding a capsule or a gel cap to that existing stash of medications is easy enough, so start there. Lower doses seem preferable to make sure there are no interactions, so starting even lower and even slower than I outline elsewhere in the book may be wise. There's no harm or shame in starting with a smaller amount, such as five milligrams over five days, to test the waters. If that dose seems safe but ineffective, double it over the same duration and then revaluate. Secondarily, as anxiety comes up, and exasperates other symptoms of pain and sleeplessness, consider up-dosing.

The initial dose you start to take for inflammation may well alleviate some concerns around anxiety, pain, and sleeplessness. If it doesn't, adding something a little bit more localized and targeted may offer relief. For example, depending on where your pain presents, a topical additive may feel quite good. (Flip to Chapter 7 for more on topicals.) Anxiety often seems to require a higher dose, but I also strongly believe that anxiety and inflammation are linked. I think that if you create a ritual around consumption for inflammation relief, then you're also promoting overall remediation. You may not need something stronger.

TIP

The Sagely brand has a great variety of inflammation-specific products, and they're quite widely available. I tend to be partial to the company's roll-on applicator because it's easy to use and provides its own little massage in the process. They're available on walmart.com. For a little more upscale and fun version of a pain relief roll-on, check out Tonic brand, available on the company's website and also through my company Poplar (www.shop-poplar.com).

TIP

If you want to start with sleep, or you just need a little something extra with all that you've already got going on, take a bath. I can't overstate how much CBD baths are a one-size-fits-all remedy — relaxing, destressing, pain-relieving, roll-right-into-bed goodness. A brand with 75 to 150 milligrams of CBD and a variety of other beautiful botanicals to make the experience smell as nice as possible will change your night, if not your life. For the added benefits of muscle and pain relief make sure the product has a good dose of magnesium and Epsom salts (see Chapter 12 for details). Rosebud brands bath salts are quite nice, and I also like the Bade Collection.

Chapter **14**

Alleviating Issues Specific to Age and Sex

As we age, we go through a plethora of psychological and physiological experiences. Many of them are good and even necessary. On the flip side, plenty of age-related experiences can use all the beneficial attention they can get. A great aspect of CBD is that it can help people of all ages and maturity levels. Its varied psychological and physiological benefits mean we may find some relief as it comes to aging.

In this chapter, I explore topical applications of CBD for supporting and slowing the appearance of aging skin. I take a deeper look at the endocannabinoid system (ECS) and specifically how it relates to women's health concerns. I also open a window into the implications of CBD as a supporting tool for both men's and women's sexual health. (*Note:* While I use these historically accepted nomenclatures to address gender, it is only because they are familiar, and current studies have not extended or explained beyond men and women and into the nonbinary community. It is very possible that sexual dysfunction across all genders may be addressed similarly with CBD.)

Addressing Skin Concerns That Coincide with Aging

Aging skin may be inevitable, but suffering doesn't have to be. Through preventative treatment and planning, you can get ahead of some of the most discouraging symptoms of skin aging. Reducing their effects allows you to be much more comfortable in the ongoing phases of your life.

One of the largest concerns about aging from a systematic level is inflammation, too much of which speeds up the aging process. You may also experience conditions that lead to internal imbalances that are more widespread.

Sagging skin and lost elasticity

Sagging skin and lost elasticity can be the result of internal damage as well as topical influences like free radicals, pollution, and other contaminants. CBD is a potent antioxidant, and it's been said that these effects can help boost collagen when combined with facial products from serums to creams. *Collagen* is responsible for the plump and often young appearance of the skin. A combination of collagen-boosting and anti-inflammatory properties may result in an overall more youthful appearance. And the advantages are noticeable. More collagen and less inflammation lead to an improved skin tone and a reduction of fine lines and wrinkles.

I highly recommend applying a regular regimen of topical CBD. You can read more about topicals in Chapter 7. Select a product that's designed specifically for anti-aging so that it contains other beneficial and complementary ingredients.

REMEMBER

The CBD isn't the only thing that's going to make the product. The reality is that a skin product itself needs to have a host of tailored, active ingredients, such as peptides, retinol, retinoids, hyaluronic acid, and vitamin C, specific to what you're looking to address. Ideally, CBD is an added benefit and support system for all those other ingredients. If CBD is the hero ingredient in a given product, that product's formulation may not be as strong as it otherwise could be. Look to brands that have a footprint in the marketplace outside of CBD; this approach makes trusting that a brand knows what it's doing from a skincare formulation standpoint a bit easier.

TIP

If you want examples of great brands for CBD skincare, check out Ildi Pekar and Khus + Khus. They have highly reviewed and established product lines in addition to a selection of distinct items that contain CBD as a complementary ingredient. Prima brand actually has a product called The Afterglow that has a combination of

CBD and hyaluronic acid that may be a great option; it's specifically designed for anti-aging, elasticity, and dryness.

To take this discussion one step further, think about what you're doing in conjunction with the CBD skincare you're using. Elasticity starts from the inside. A really good collagen supplement can be a great boost; look for organic and non-GMO quality sourcing. Some options are even vegan.

Scar tissue

Scar tissue contributes heavily to the appearance and physical discomfort associated with scars. Though the physical appearance of scars may not necessarily be desirable, one of the most negative aspects of scarring is the potential pain associated with scar tissue buildup from an injury. Reducing that scar tissue can actually be a quite painful process. It often requires outside tools or heavy and steady pressure with someone's hand.

The pain-relieving effects of topical CBD may help remediate some of that pain during the process of working out the scar tissue. This all depends on the amount of affected surface area and how old or painful the scar tissue is. Taking internal CBD should also help because it addresses the anti-inflammatory process from an internal perspective. Increasing blood flow by reducing inflammation may help fade the appearance of scars. Couple that with a massage style application of some topical CBD, and you're also doing wonders for your skin. You're not only increasing microcirculation but also breaking up scar tissue.

It has also been said that the application of CBD may support or even boost the healing time of scars. Early studies are starting to show evidence that CBD is supporting cell turnover. Couple the cell turnover with collagen-boosting properties, and you may just have a solution to fade scars. Currently, studies are seeing acne patients with positive results.

Clearing up Acne and Other Conditions

Early research has indicated CBD's potential ability to decrease excess oil (sebum) production in the skin. The result is a positive balancing effect. Combine that ability with the overall anti-inflammatory effects, and CBD can prove to be helpful for treating skin conditions topically. Its antifungal, antibacterial, and antimicrobial effects may also be beneficial here.

Addressing acne

Acne is very common in people of various ages and sexes, so it has been deeply studied. While acne is most often associated as a teen problem or condition, there is, in fact, a prevalence of adult acne on par with teen acne. That said, adult acne is more common in women. Acne is an inflammatory condition, and information exists to suggest it has internal triggers. Anti-inflammatory topicals are said to provide a soothing sensation and reduce redness related to breakouts.

Beyond that, CBD's antibacterial, antimicrobial, and antifungal properties may prove to be incredibly beneficial for specific types of acne. For example, acne flare-ups that are induced by topical agitators such as free radicals are definite candidates for CBD, as are congestion in the skin from dirt and bacterial interactions. In these particular situations, cleaning the skin topically is probably the best bet for prevention. However, during active breakouts, applying cleansers with anti-inflammatory and antibacterial properties is probably a good idea. This benefit is why CBD skincare is a win-win for acne.

Reducing rosacea

Rosacea is another common skin condition that causes redness and sometimes increased visibility of blood vessels in the face. The redness can persist, creating not only an unwanted appearance but also sometimes additional discomfort. Rosacea is skin stress that can be caused by internal stressors such as food sensitivity — including alcohol — but also triggered by external ones such as hairspray (yes, hairspray) and pollution.

All information points to the fact that the soothing effects of CBD can be very beneficial in treating outbreaks of rosacea. But internal and topical use of CBD products have also been shown to potentially help combat some of the internal causes and prevent outbreaks altogether. So my advice is simple: Lean on the anti-inflammatory benefits of CBD and recognize that a two-pronged approach of internal tinctures and topical applications may be the best remedy for the primary and secondary symptoms of your rosacea.

TIP

Paula's Choice Skincare has a CBD Oil + Retinol that can be used for rosacea. It's specifically designed for tough cases with frequent flare-ups. Retinol in conjunction with CBD digs deep to address the underlying causes of roseacea. This type of product is also great to counteract some of the signs of aging, like fine lines and wrinkles. Flip to the section "Addressing Skin Concerns That Coincide with Aging" earlier in the chapter for more on using CBD to combat the signs of aging.

Eliminating eczema

Eczema, much like rosacea (see the preceding section), is a skin condition that causes red, inflamed, rash-like, and potentially even itchy skin. Mild manifestations of this condition can appear almost like dry skin. But when it goes untreated, it'll likely worsen. A less common form of eczema is called *atopic*. It's a result of a minimized (and therefore more sensitive/reactive) natural skin barrier, so it's more common in children and something they may grow out of over time.

Eczema is said to be a reaction to allergens like food, pet dander, pollens, and chemicals found in everyday materials, including fabrics. Most flare-ups in the eczema family are related to exposure to triggers. CBD is proving to be a promising treatment for eczema because of its ability to decrease itching and pain induced by inflammation.

CBD for eczema should be a really simple, clear formulation with no irritants that may amplify the condition. Some would go so far as to say the cleanest and most efficient way to treat eczema with CBD is a water-based product because an oil base can congest the skin and prevent cell turnover. The point is that sensitivity is high with eczema, and ingredients in skincare products treating it should be designed to be soothing. Coconut oil is a cooling oil. Sunflower oil and calendula are both said to be beneficial for eczema.

TIP

The brand The Alchemist's Kitchen has a calming calendula face oil that has all the right ingredients. I haven't tried the brand, but it has been a go-to for naturalists for a long time, and I certainly consider them trustworthy. As a lovely bonus, the product has some of the calming benefits needed to treat acne flare-ups as well (see the earlier section "Addressing acne" for more).

Answering common CBD skincare questions

The most common question is, "Why would you use CBD for skin?" As an anti-inflammatory, antibacterial, and antimicrobial, it has so many beneficial qualities. Skin issues can be due to aging caused by exposure to pollutants and free radicals, as well as inflammation. This means CBD is the perfect ally. In this section, I answer other common questions about products, pollution, and more!

What if I live in an area with poor air quality and my breakouts are due to pollutants and smog?

You may wonder where to start if you're worried about acne congestion and buildup on the skin. Those living in smog-heavy areas should be practicing a very thorough skincare regimen to not only keep their skin clean but also protect it. In this case, CBD makes a lot of sense because it has an incredible combination of cleansing, preventative, reparative, and protective capabilities.

The first step in treating pollution-related breakouts and skin congestion is a really good cleanser. The truth about CBD and cleansers is they're not necessarily a good combination. Ideally, cleansers gently remove everything that's on the skin's surface. That means whatever is in the formulation is coming off quickly thereafter. If you happen to find a cleanser that's designed to sit on the face for a longer period, then CBD as an ingredient may be justifiable. The CBD molecule is slightly larger than some, so it doesn't penetrate or absorb as easily into the top layer of the skin. Absorption is how you get the best benefits of CBD.

The CBD molecule itself is a lipid base, which means that the cleanser needs to have a fatty component or oil to even carry the CBD as an ingredient. CBD skincare cleansers should be oil-based; that way, you can be confident that the CBD is part of the formulation rather than just suspended amid the ingredients.

TIP

Verte Essentials brand makes a micellar water cleansing pad that has a combination of oil- and water-based ingredients perfect for removing makeup as well as pollutants. The pad's exfoliating properties and application style help remove grime and let the active ingredients penetrate the skin.

How do I know what to look for in CBD skincare products?

Telling the difference between what one CBD skincare line does and what another does can be tough. The truth is that I've struggled with that very task myself. Most of the brands offering CBD skincare seem to come to the market with serums rather which are oil-based topical products in a dropper vial. Sometimes they have other ingredients that seem to be active, and sometimes they don't.

A really good skincare product can have a diversity of active ingredients that complement and support one another in various ways. A basic daily skincare routine may not need a ton of active ingredients. It really just depends on what you're looking for. If you're after a specific outcome, however, identifying which key ingredients will support your needs is important. The preceding sections on various skin conditions can help point you in the right direction on that front.

REMEMBER

It really is too early in the CBD skincare game for the competitive marketplace to have a large variety of products with good active formulations. But the active benefits of CBD are so broad. If you have an untreated or poorly treated skincare condition, you may find great relief from any simple addition of CBD to your regimen, even if the product market isn't perfect at this exact moment.

CBD OFFERS A WELCOME FOCUS ON WOMEN'S HEALTH

Here's a fun fact: The *endocannabinoid system* (the body's internal cannabinoid system, which consists of CB1 and CB2 receptors and a host of enzymes) expresses a really high concentration of these receptors in the uterus. The second highest concentration of receptors in the ECS is found in the pelvic region — second only to the brain.

CBD is starting to appear in every sort of women's health product, and for good reason: Many women's health conditions include inflammation and pain. Sexism in the science industry has rendered many prominent women's health conditions invisible from an informational standpoint. Female health issues have been severely understudied for generations, so the opportunity to find relief and benefits in new forms is enthusiastically welcomed.

If a product from a beauty retailer contains cannabis sativa seed oil or hemp seed oil, does that mean it has CBD oil?

REMEMBER

To be clear, neither hemp seed oil nor cannabis sativa seed oil is interchangeable with CBD. The seeds of the plant are protein-based, and they're amazing for consumption and digestion. However, they don't contain CBD. Though using these oils topically does have other benefits, the oils aren't the same as CBD oil.

The confusion began in part because when many beauty stores wanted to get into carrying CBD, they were met with legal obstacles. Navigating the legal gray area meant they were prevented from carrying actual CBD, so they picked up brands that were using hemp seed oil or cannabis sativa seed oil.

Relieving Menstrual Cramps

Menstrual cramps, or *dysmenorrhea*, are the cramping pain before, during, and after a woman's menstrual cycle. Though some women don't experience any sensation at all, others can have incredibly debilitating pain. The sensations are caused by the production of *prostaglandin*, a chemical to help the muscles of the uterus contract and consequently push blood out of the system. External triggers like stress can lead to an overproduction of prostaglandin released from the uterine lining, which results in correspondingly intense physical cramps.

Because the anti-inflammatory properties of CBD result in the sensation of pain relief, internal use of CBD during a woman's menstrual cycle is showing to have positive effects such as the reduction of cramping and associated pain. Topical applications of CBD creams and balms have been touted for their ability to soothe cramps, but their relief may be temporary or not as deeply effective.

TIP

Prostaglandin overproduction may also be due to an imbalance in the system. Full-spectrum CBD used internally may help with overall balance *(homeostasis)*. It may help get the prostaglandin in check, creating a balance in the system and offering deeper, longer-lasting relief rather than just creating pain relief opportunities.

Suppositories

As I mention in the earlier sidebar, there are a huge amount of receptors for cannabis in the pelvic region, and therefore that area of the body is going to be particularly receptive to CBD medicine. While many forms get CBD into the bloodstream, nothing is quite like a suppository.

The rise of CBD suppositories is something to pay attention to. More and more are coming to the market because, frankly, they work. The United States has been slow to adopt the suppository form factor for medicine delivery, but the rest of the world has been using it for generations.

The reason this delivery method is so great is that this region of the body has a lot of receptors, so you can deliver an incredible amount of medicine without the unintended side effects of high doses. Both vaginal and rectal insertion are options here. The formulation behind these suppositories doesn't vary much from brand to brand. It usually consists of a base of coconut oil and a high concentration of full-spectrum CBD extract. I recommend 50 milligrams as the baseline to see major relief from cramps.

One of the first and foremost brands on the market was Foria, known known for addressing women's health and feminine sexual pleasure. Another brand, IYP (In Your Pleasure), is new to the market. It has added an additional spin to its suppository with the boost of magnesium. Magnesium's role is to help relax muscles and to loosen the tissue. These jobs are key in addressing menstrual cramps. Because so many people are magnesium-deficient, this product creates a great complementary pairing. If these aren't doing the trick and you think you might need a boost with THC (and you live in a place where you can access it legally), companies like Hello Again are creating some great like-minded suppositories with THC. And you can rest easy knowing the THC, when used regionally in these doses, isn't going to get you high.

TECHNICAL
STUFF

The reason for the name IYP is deeply intuitive. Suppositories there are not only good for pain relief but also great for pleasure. Some people have uncomfortable sex or cramps during sex for any of a number of reasons. So if a suppository can address both lower abdomen cramping and sexual discomfort, then it seems like a win-win.

TIP

I know the thought of using a suppository is uncomfortable to many, but then again, so are painful cramps. To make the application feel a little less unusual, Amazon carries disposable suppository applicators. For tampon-users, this tool lends a level of familiarity. If you're not a fan of single-use plastic disposals or unnecessary devices, know that the brand IYP has plans to release a reusable stylish copper applicator. Copper is not only beautiful, but it also has a long healing history for women's health across cultures.

Transdermal patches

Transdermal patches are also extremely beneficial; such patches applied to the lower back region can have a heating and cooling sensation while delivering CBD directly into the bloodstream. If you've ever used a traditional Chinese medicine pain patch, it's much the same sensation, but with the added benefits of CBD's pain relief. Chapter 7 has more on transdermal patches.

TIP

Mary's Nutritionals has one of the most trusted CBD transdermal patches on the market. It's not specifically designed for menstrual cramps, but you can use it for them by placing it on either side of your lower back or on top of your pelvis.

The marketing for a product by La Mend called The Good Patch suggests it may combat symptoms of PMS, though the product looks a little less targeted than others I mention.

Bath soaks

A really amazing CBD soak is a surefire ticket for relief. Designed properly, it has a variety of other complementary ingredients to deliver just what your body needs. For example, a soak for cramps may include magnesium to address muscle tension, chamomile to calm nerves, lavender to decompress the nervous system, and additional mineral salts to replenish mineral deficiencies. Also, baking soda (sodium bicarbonate) is often present to absorb any toxins released into the tub while soaking. While the baking soda is not necessary for the relief of cramps, it will help absorb toxins. When your body is out of balance, anything you can do to help restore that state of balance is important so that your body is not working in overdrive to address a particular condition. And of course CBD is the holy grail for deep relaxation and inflammation relief.

TIP

A few of my favorite products are the Peace of Mind Soak by Verte Essentials, Vertly Soak Bath Salts, and Empower Bodycare's collection, all of which are available on www.shop-poplar.com/.

WARNING

Don't confuse a bath soak with a bath bomb. Bath bombs are nice for a good relaxing soak, but they don't contain nearly the array of minerals and botanicals needed to fully address severe cramps.

Teas and balms

Two other products for addressing cramping are teas and balms.

REMEMBER

These options largely hold their tradition in the comfort of ritual because their benefits are somewhat limited in terms of *bioavailability* (your body's ability to absorb the ingredients). Getting CBD into the bloodstream is crucial for beginning to address internal pain and muscular cramping of this nature. A tea must go through the digestive tract, which makes the CBD and other ingredients less available to your bloodstream. A balm is any CBD-based topical that has a thicker consistency than a lotion and requires a heavier hand to massage it into the skin. One of the added benefits of a balm is the massaging technique of application stimulates microcirculation under the skin, which is great for blood flow and circulation. It is not, however, transdermal in nature.

With the right ingredients, however, these products potentially have other benefits. A great combination is hemp and *nervines,* which are botanicals that support the healthy function of the nervous system and ultimately decompress an elevated or imbalanced system. These ingredients include chamomile and lavender, which are common in calming teas. So choose a tea that has hemp and either of these two ingredients, or make the right nervine tea and add your CBD tincture.

Considering CBD during Pregnancy and Breastfeeding

This topic carries a ton of controversy with it, largely because of the history of cannabis and hemp as controlled substances in the United States. Most Western medical experts and the FDA will tell you CBD and anything related to cannabis are a no-go.

You must know the laws in your state (that is, the state where you plan on delivering and raising your child). Even though some hemp-derived CBD has been declassified since 2018, the prohibition mindset still exists, and not all states are beyond prosecuting minor infractions. In some states, authorities can still remove your child from your custody if they find concentrations of THC in your system. According to the medical system in states with laws prohibiting cannabis and CBD, they would only test a new mother in a hospital should they be given cause. However, I have yet to see that written anywhere in stone. Chapter 6 has information on various state regulations regarding CBD and THC, but be sure to investigate your state's current guidelines on these chemicals and parenting specifically. It is also worth noting that testing has been designed to check for concentrations of THC, not CBD. That said, some CBD products, most full- and broad-spectrum, will contain a small amount of THC, so it's possible that THC could show up on a drug test.

Cannabis and pregnancy

The majority of research surrounding cannabis use and pregnancy has been done on THC specifically and not on CBD.

If you do a little digging, you'll find that most of the studies indicate that cannabis use had no adverse side effects on pregnancy. The concern is ultimately that cannabis use may compromise the neurological development of a baby in the womb. Consider, though, that the U.S. government has a patent on non-psychoactive cannabis, including CBD, to protect the brain from damage or degeneration. This designation is a direct claim that cannabis is neuroprotective.

Studies have indicated human cannabinoids and cannabinoid receptors have an important influence in prenatal and post-natal development. As I previously mention, the body is full of cannabinoid receptors. For example, the presence of CB1 receptors has been detected in the pre- and post-natal nervous system, suggesting an important and intrinsic link to brain development. Anandamide, the endocannabinoid known as the bliss molecule, is also prevalent in the embryo and uterus pre-implantation. This research hasn't been further developed in any consumer-facing way since the early 2000s, but it's only a matter of time.

So many aspects of the physical experience of being pregnant are new to the body and, frankly, often uncomfortable. Muscle pain, fatigue, nausea, sleeplessness, brain fog, stress, and general discomfort are just some of them. On a positive note, CBD has been recognized to address most if not all of them.

I live in a state with very strict regulations, but I consumed CBD during my entire pregnancy. It came from a hemp–derived, isolate source, so no THC was present in my system. (Chapter 7 has more on isolate.) I do — and did then — know a fair amount on the subject, and I was consuming CBD long before my child was conceived. Knowing my dose and what worked for me when, where, and how was an important part of using CBD as a medicine and a tool for relief.

If you decide to go this route, slow and low is the technique of choice; see Chapter 5. The less distress you're in, the fewer complications and discomforts are present in your pregnancy experience.

AFFECTING BREASTMILK WITH CBD

In late 2019, I embarked on a private study on breast milk and CBD. Because there were no existing studies at the time to indicate what was safe and what was actually beneficial. The study began with me. Because I've been in the CBD space for so long, I know countless women who have consumed cannabis containing THC and CBD long before, during, and after having a baby. I've also read everything I can get my hands on about the history of cannabis in ancient practices and other cultures. This research provided me with the security I needed to be my own guinea pig.

Throughout my pregnancy, I consumed CBD cannabis in various forms. When my son was born, I stopped consuming any form of CBD merely to test the natural concentration of endocannabinoids in my milk without supplementation. The purpose of this experiment was to create a baseline. Sad to say, when the time came to test my milk for natural endocannabinoids, my supply was starting to dry up. And circumstances weren't ideal; the potential to test my milk again later with supplemental CBD wasn't going to be an option. So the study is shelved for now.

I came to this study because in testing, natural endocannabinoids in breast milk have shown the presence of anandamide. Anandamide, otherwise known as the bliss molecule, plays a role in feeding regulation as well as pleasure and motivation. The bliss response keeps a baby feeding. The other, most dominant endocannabinoid found in babies is 2-arachidonoylglycerol, or 2-AG. Unsurprisingly, it's a sweet-tasting, androgynous internal cannabinoid that interacts with the CB1 receptors in the brain, controlling the suckling response and tongue muscles. Sweet, huh? Maybe that's part of the flavor of breast milk!

CBD and breastfeeding

I believe that a bit of CBD in your milk supply isn't the worst thing. I've come to this conclusion with quite a bit of support:

>> The U.S. government has deemed cannabinoids — like CBD — neuroprotective.

>> The human body is naturally filled with cannabinoids. Some of these endocannabinoids have been detected in the milk of nursing mothers.

>> The trend toward general relief without side effects from supplemental CBD use is incredibly promising.

The only real study to date tracking cannabinoid transmission into milk supply was done on THC. Only 2.5 percent of the mother's THC intake was transferred to the milk. The study didn't include CBD, nor did it probe further to determine whether the THC had actually transferred into the babies' bodies.

CAN CBD EASE THE EFFECTS OF HORMONE IMBALANCES?

Hormones are message-delivering chemicals produced in the endocrine system. They travel throughout the body regulating most major processes, such as metabolism, reproductive cycles, mood and stress, body temperature, and even sleep cycles. A misfire in any of these hormonal systems can trigger results ranging from mood and mental health issues to sexual dysfunction and infertility to skin, blood pressure, and pain issues, to name just a few. (When I said they address most bodily functions, I wasn't kidding.)

CBD's applications for supporting a variety of bodily functions, and especially its anti-inflammatory properties, seem to indicate some degree of opportunity to address the symptoms of hormonal imbalances. But whether it can help remediate the imbalances themselves is another question. Because CBD is touted for its ability to help balance the system (cannabis specifically is noted for its ability to create homeostasis), CBD very well may be an important piece in addressing hormonal balance at a core level.

What does transfer into the babies' bodies through the milk supply is cortisol. *Cortisol* is a stress hormone that prepares you to feel alarmed or fearful. Apparently, babies are highly sensitive to cortisol. Infants take all of their cues from their mothers energetically, emotionally, and physiologically. In my experience, my baby was highly sensitive to anything I was feeling. CBD has been shown to prevent the overflow of cortisol, so I'd personally much rather take CBD to mitigate my stress, knowing that any CBD my child may get in the milk supply will protect from excessive amounts of cortisol.

Making Menopause Bearable

Menopause is a life stage marked by hormonal changes in the female body due to age. From what I understand, there are few changes associated with menopause that are desirable. Table 14-1 outlines and separates the common menopause symptoms and how CBD might be able to help. Additionally, I break out some of the other, really unpleasant side effects that can actually contribute to exasperating other symptoms, such as anxiety and sleeplessness as well as painful sex and libido changes.

TABLE 14-1 **Treating Menopause Symptoms with CBD**

Common Symptoms of Menopause	How Can CBD Specifically Help?
Weight gain and slowed metabolism	CBD can improve sleep patterns, helping to reduce anxiety, and mitigating stress hormone dysfunction associated with metabolism. In this way, an overall balance may be achieved to help prevent weight gain.
Night sweats	CBD hasn't yet been shown to mitigate night sweats. But it certainly has been indicated as capable of helping with sleep. With deep and thorough enough rest, maybe the night sweats won't wake you up.
Breast soreness	Because of CBD's pain-relieving properties, an ingestible tincture or some good old balm may relieve some of this tenderness.
Hair loss	For some, hair loss at this stage in life is related to stress and the discomfort associated with other symptoms. CBD may help mitigate the stress.

STRESS INCONTINENCE

Stress incontinence (where even small movements or actions put pressure on the bladder and make you go a little) is ultimately caused by a weakening of the pelvic floor. In fact, although stress incontinence is timed with menopause, for many it can actually just be a symptom of aging and decreased muscle tone. A healthy routine of pelvic floor exercises like Kegels can really help. Additionally, yoga is excellent for strengthening the pelvic floor.

Other reported symptoms of menopause include

>> **Anxiety and bouts of sleeplessness:** These symptoms tend to be the most commonly reported and the most beneficially remediated with CBD. Studies have indicated across human use that CBD can reduce perceptions of anxiety and stress as well as depression. CBD has also been indicated to promote better sleep.

>> **Joint pain.**

>> **Mood imbalances.**

>> **Vaginal dryness and painful sex:** Topical CBD and sometimes even CBD suppositories, which are becoming more and more popular, can address these concerns. Head to the earlier section "Suppositories" for more on this option.

REMEMBER

Few side effects have been reported from using CBD to relieve these symptoms. This low level is not so much the case with traditional medicines used to remedy menopausal effects.

Black cohosh is one of the most studied botanicals to treat symptoms of menopause, especially hot flashes. Some studies indicate that it can help tremendously. However, it's not recommended for those taking medications that require processing through the liver, or people with any sort of liver problems at all. Because of this, some CBD treatments are designed with black cohosh with the intent of addressing hot flashes. THC is more widely recognized as a cannabinoid that can address temperature changes, but CBD is more widely available, and thus evolution in CBD products is imminent.

TIP

The only product with the combination of these two ingredients I've seen to date is Menopause Relief Oil from the brand Dr. Evans. It is formulated by a doctor who's always been focused on the women's health space.

Helping with Sexual Dysfunction Issues

Sexual dysfunction is broadly defined as not experiencing pleasure during sex. If pain or anxiety is getting in the way, CBD is absolutely your friend. If it's a matter of mood, CBD may be there to hold your hand as well. And rightfully so, there is little pleasure to be had if erectile dysfunction (ED) is an issue. If ED is caused by blood flow, anxiety, or mood issues, CBD could help you men out too.

Lifting your libido

Your *libido* is actually your sex drive or your desire to engage in sexual activity. Sex drive can actually be affected by myriad causes, from psychological factors to general lack of pleasure to physical discomfort or even serious pain.

Little research indicates that CBD itself actually boosts the libido. Some opinions even suggest that it does the opposite. More evidence exists to suggest that a combination of CBD and THC is most beneficial in supporting the libido.

The female libido is quite multifaceted. It fluctuates over the years with hormonal changes and mood changes around major life events, such as changes in relationships, depression, and the stresses of age. A lot of sexual dysfunction is associated with pain that no doubt compromises the desire or pleasure found in a sexual experience; you can read more about CBD for vaginal pain issues in the following section.

CBD mostly helps with libido by getting you out of your own way in order to experience an increased interest in pleasure. If stress is the culprit, the right dose of CBD may be effective in addressing negative libido changes. I simply recommend CBD supplementation and an everyday product like a sublingual or an edible in doses ranging from 10 to 30 milligrams once or twice a day depending on your need. If the thought of sexual activity is what's causing the stress, you may consider consuming a higher dose before foreplay. Good forms for this approach may include smoking or inhalation for the quick onset time or consuming an edible 30 minutes or so before activity.

If mood is more at the root of the issue, complement your CBD use with some cacao. Cacao is known to boost or supplement natural anandamide levels; you can read more about anandamide earlier in the chapter and in Chapter 2. The Western medical system tends to prescribe mood-enhancing drugs here, but these tend to have somewhat of a numbing effect in all regards.

TIP

My recommendation is to go straight for Calivolve chocolate bar. This brand even has a bar specifically designed for arousal and intimacy. Foria, a brand driven by sex and pleasure, also has a cool product called Awaken for enhancing libido.

Rising to the occasion (so to speak)

When it comes to *erectile dysfunction* (ED), chronic health conditions and generally poor self-care can contribute to the issue. Often caused by anxiety and mood conditions (both of which can be addressed with CBD), there is hope in addressing ED. A supplemental form, taken on a regular basis to balance out mood or eliminate anxiety, may be an option. In this instance, I would suggest an easy-to-take format that can be incorporated into an existing routine, like gel capsules or a tincture one to two times a day. However, it could be just a quick blast of CBD in the moment to relieve some anxiety, in which case I would recommend a fast-acting form, like a vape pen or other smokable.

For ED caused by potential inflammation or restricted blood flow, smoking, over time, diminishes blood flow. Alcohol likewise can cause ED. Other chronic health conditions that create changes in blood flow, such as diabetes, can also be the cause. Theories suggest that CBD can help with blood flow, particularly if it is compromised via inflammation. Again, I would recommend supplements for an overall and longer-term relief, and fast-acting in the moment, for, well, exactly that.

Preventing vaginal pain

Because of CBD's anti-inflammatory properties and its suggested pain relief response, the potential for using it for relieving sexual pain is a no-brainer. Less pain means an increase in sexual pleasure.

Vaginal pain may be the result of uterine fibroids or vaginal dryness. In cases where you want less friction, why not use a lubricant that contains CBD? As I mention earlier in the chapter, the uterus has an incredible number of CB1 receptors. This pre-existing framework indicates that your responses and benefits may be high.

Increasing sensation

Reducing inflammation in the body and throughout the system also helps increase blood flow to tissues. The end result is an increase in sensitivity. I won't get into the intimate details, but you catch my drift. Regional topicals and internal dosing can each increase sensitivity. Each method can have similar intended benefits so long as you're paying attention to onset time; topicals have a shorter onset than internal forms.

TIP

The CBD marketplace has no shortage of arousal oils. These products intend to do more than a traditional lubricant by virtue of CBD's potential benefits of decreasing stress, increasing blood flow and stimulation, and decreasing pain. Foria is the leader in this space with a wide selection of products. Its Awaken Arousal Oil is a great starting point, or it also has a starter set called the Quickie Kit. You can locate its products on its website and many other third-party websites.

Another new really fun and cool brand that helps with all of my favorite things, from sustainability to inclusivity, is called WLDKAT. It has a prebiotic and pH-balanced sex serum that serves as not only a lube but also a revitalizer. The prebiotic aspect helps balance bacteria and keep your body healthy. This lube is also water-based. The benefit of a water-based formulation is that you can use it with latex condoms, which for some is a necessity with partner play. Many CBD lubricants on the market are oil-based, and latex condoms don't play well with oil. This product is available on the brand's website, https://wldkat.com/.

IN THIS CHAPTER

» Getting familiar with the CBD use in pets

» Helping pets with anxiety and PTSD

» Calming cancer symptoms and treatment side effects

» Using CBD for dogs with seizure issues and epilepsy

» Making sure you're giving the correct dosage and watching out for adverse reactions

Chapter 15

Letting Pets Benefit from CBD

With the overwhelming evidence that CBD is helping myriad human ailments, deducing that pets may find benefits for what ails them as well seems only logical. The language barrier may present a challenge, but various signals from your animal's behavior can help you figure out whether CBD is genuinely helping them.

This chapter explores how CBD may help your pets by exploring the multiple conditions they may suffer from, including anxiety in various forms, cancer, PTSD, and weak appetites. You also get helpful guidance on dosing and spotting potential adverse reactions.

Determining How CBD May Help Your Pet

Your pets may not be *Homo sapiens*, but they're still your homies. They suffer from many of the same conditions humans do. Pets are one of the largest financially attractive markets in the United States; profit and personal attachment have led companies and individuals to want to provide pets with the healthiest benefits available. Particularly, those who prefer the most natural solutions have a similar desire to support their furry and feathered family members with the same consideration level. If you're wondering whether and how your pet may benefit from CBD, this section gets you started with the basics.

You may also be wondering what kind of pet I might be talking about here. I do lean heavily into dogs, with a bit of info on cats. The truth is most CBD studies have been done on rodents, so most of what you see applied here, and across the whole book for that matter, might just apply to your rodent pets. But as with all animals, calculating the dose based on the weight of your pet is maybe the single most important part to this puzzle. CBD is becoming quite popular in the equine market as well, but I don't drive us in that direction because that is an industry of sport all in itself — again, weight matters, and there are plenty of form factors out there available specifically for the equine market. For all other pets, consider size — and know that you may be taking some risks, as not much has been done by way of study on our lizard pets, goldfish, or parakeets.

Asking the right questions

Though CBD holds limitless potential for symptom reduction in humans, pet owners and veterinarians alike have a healthy amount of distrust about whether CBD is ideal for animals. Human consumption is generally the research priority, and even that research is still in the early stages. Far less CBD research exists specifically around pet friends and whether CBD can benefit them.

REMEMBER

Although there isn't much yet in the way of pet research specifically, research is abundant in the animal space overall because clinical trials almost always begin in animal models. Most technical analysis in the CBD space, basically as an industry standard, is on rodents. Mice may not be common pets, but they're more akin to your furry friends, biologically and physiologically, than humans are.

Here are explanations for the two most common questions:

>> **Is CBD toxic for my beloved pet?** CBD in its natural form is indicated as safe and well-tolerated. If you have a pet with severe plant allergies, you may want to use caution the first time or two to make sure they don't have any allergic

reactions. Pet friends can have liver interactions much like humans can, which requires mindfulness. If you have an animal already presenting with liver conditions or diseases that require medications processed through the liver, it might be safer to steer clear. But ask your vet.

>> **Will CBD get my pet high?** CBD available on the wide-open national marketplace, be it for pets or humans, still must adhere to the same guidelines of 0.3 percent THC or less. A level of THC this low won't get a human high, nor will it induce a high in your pet. Head to Chapter 6 for more on the CBD marketplace in general and on the laws regarding THC.

Check the label to make sure it indicates the proper levels of THC. The pet space doesn't have less regulation, but in general, tracking down anecdotal evidence is probably a little bit harder here than it is for CBD intended for people.

Reviewing conditions that CBD may help alleviate

CBD is advantageous for humans, pets, you name it. Just like in humans, inflammation is often at the source of what ails animals.

CBD is most commonly used to help manage the following conditions in pets:

>> **Anxiety:** Anxiety may have compounded effects in pets that have a lot of stressors in their environments. They, of course, can't say, "Hey, I'm stressed out!" This inability to communicate can lead pets to suffer from perpetual anxious feelings. With so many people adopting pets from third parties and adoption centers, post-traumatic stress disorder (PTSD) becomes more common in pets from these backgrounds. The variety of products on the marketplace provides the opportunity to find the right dose of CBD that may give your animal friends anxiety relief as well.

>> **Cancer:** To date, nothing leads researchers to believe that CBD is a cancer cure. However, it can very well help you address symptoms associated with your pet's cancer and cancer treatments, including loss of appetite, stress, and sleep challenges. As well, an overall reduction in inflammation can prove to be beneficial.

>> **Seizures:** The first and only FDA-approved CBD product on the legal pharmaceutical marketplace for humans is Epidiolex, which is an anti-seizure medication. With this knowledge, and the similarities between humans' and animals' chemistry, pet owners use CBD to help diminish seizures or the side effects of these unfortunate neurological episodes. Epidiolex isn't made for our pet friends, so I only bring it up to encourage you to embrace CBD as a seizure medication.

Note: I cover each of these conditions and CBD treatments for them in more detail in the following three sections.

Aiding an Anxious Pet

The manifestations of pet anxiety can appear in nearly endless ways:

>> Destructive behaviors that are often dismissed as bad behavior, such as decimating furniture, beds, and car seats

>> Self-directed or external aggression

>> Urination and defecation in the house or in different zones that are "their" space

>> Excessive drooling and panting

>> Excessive barking and pacing or even exaggerating normal reactionary behavior to an incident

Other characteristics like digging, body posture changes, and even changes in bodily functions can be symptoms of stress. In mellow and easygoing pets, these are all signs of anxiety. Getting a sense of what your pet is exhibiting as anxiety is essential.

Though pet lovers have found ways to relieve anxiety in their furry friends, from quality time to introducing another companion to taking multiple daily walks, animals still suffer from anxiety. This section looks at some different ways CBD can help with different sources of anxiety.

REMEMBER

The size discrepancy between animals and humans requires a more in-depth examination of the dosing requirements necessary to aid anxiety relief. Numerous products on the marketplace are designed specifically for pets highlight the poundage to dosage ratio required to address these considerations. I also discuss dosing calculations in the later section "Getting Good with Dosing."

Soothing stress from separation

Because the pet market is so large, many tools, devices, and training techniques are available to pet owners to help in *decompression* (that is, decompressing the nervous system to make an animal feel safe). For stress from separation anxiety, some tools include compression blankets and weighted blankets. Animals use toys as outlets for their stress, whether that plays out as snuggling with or ripping apart their plush pet accessories. Some pet owners have found that providing a well-used personal item to their pet while they're apart offers scent association and, in turn, comfort.

With CBD, you can give your animal some treats and tinctures directly or add them to treats. Some treats and dog foods contain hemp proteins to help support a dog's overall immune function holistically with the full spectrum of hemp. (Chapter 2 has more on hemp.) Just like in humans, tinctures and oils are going to have more fast-acting benefits than a consumable like a dog treat.

TIP

Here are a couple of product suggestions:

>> Sometimes getting a dog (or any other animal, for that matter) to take a tincture can be hard. That's why brands like Terra Vita have created animal products with more desirable flavors like bacon. The Half Day CBD brand was generous enough to share a recipe for something that you can make at home (check the Pumpkin and Peanut Butter dog treats in Chapter 18).

>> Holistapet offers pet treats specifically for dogs with stress and anxiety. They're also healthy, so they make an excellent option for knowing you're treating every part of your dog well. These types of remedies are likely best served up just post-tincture if you're going away for several hours and want to make sure your pet is taken care of for the whole time you're gone.

Treating anxiety in dogs with PTSD

PTSD can be a little bit trickier than treating separation anxiety (see the preceding section). It's a whole different animal, so to speak. It can require higher doses of CBD and sometimes in different forms to make sure you're covering durations.

PTSD symptoms in your animal may appear similar to severe anxiety, but events, such as loud noises, may trigger the onset of symptoms. My dog has PTSD. We got her at the shelter when she was only four months old. She seemed like a typical happy pup, with love, energy, and joy in her system. We took her on a hike one day, where she heard a gunshot far off in the distance, likely from somebody hunting. She reacted by running as fast as she could, back to what she thought was the safest space. We found her at the trailhead, cowering under the wheel of our truck, shaking uncontrollably. Even with our presence and cuddles, we had hard time consoling her.

We don't know much about her experiences in her earliest days, so we can't say what may have occurred to create these reactions. But without a shadow of a doubt, we know now that loud noises — from gunshots to fireworks to a misfiring muffler — send her nervous system into flight mode. For these sorts of reactions, if she'll take it, a tincture is best, but a treat will do if she's a little too out of it for us to put a tincture in her mouth.

More potent doses are required for these types of symptoms, so go with half a milligram for every pound of body weight:

Weight in pounds × 0.5 milligrams = Dose size in milligrams

So a 50-pound pet requires 25 milligrams of CBD for severe symptoms such as those from PTSD. Dosing is lower for a standardized regular dose, as I explain in the later section "Starting low."

Additionally, it is worth considering that a dog on a regular supplemental dose, under certain circumstances, might need an extra dose for support. For instance, a dog with severe anxiety and PTSD on a supplemental regimen might benefit from an additional serving the night of the 4th of July in the U.S. to calm any firework jitters.

Trying CBD as a Cancer Treatment

CBD isn't yet a cancer treatment per se; however, it may be a treatment for cancer's side effects. I like to look at it as an opportunity to maintain a better quality of life for your pet friends while they're suffering from a life-threatening disease. Pain, fatigue, and nausea are the more common side effects of cancer.

Shrinking tumors

Recent studies on CBD suggest that it may potentially help shrink tumors. Specifically, in pancreatic cancer, CBD illustrated a reduction in the growth of tumors and their invasive characteristics and sped up the elimination of tumors. Another study, specifically on cultured human and canine cells, found CBD beneficial in addressing *glioblastoma*, a brain cancer with malignant tumors.

CBD AND CANCER APOPTOSIS

Cancer is technically a loss of control or balance in apoptosis. *Apoptosis* is a process responsible for maintaining balance in and across cells. It essentially kills and removes unnecessary cells, which can include viral-infected or pre-cancerous cells. If this process glitches and a cancerous cell escapes, that cell can multiply in the body. This proliferation, or rather overgrowth, of cells creates malignant and/or benign tumors. CBD has been recognized as interfering with the growth, travel, and adhesion patterns of cancer cells. Because CBD has anti-tumor and anti-proliferation properties, it has a clear connection to impeding the process of cancer development.

Beyond this finding, the researchers also found that patients treated with CBD rather than a more traditional chemotherapy medication had a higher quality of life. Pain, fatigue, and nausea are often side effects of chemotherapy treatment. CBD-based treatments are an excellent vehicle for providing pain relief, soothing nausea, and supporting better rest. Feeling better overall is a reflection of a patient's immune strength, potentially indicating that the body itself is more capable of resisting the disease and fighting back alongside medicines. Studies also show that feeling good and having a will to live contribute to longevity.

REMEMBER

Studies in this area still have a long way to go. Though they indicate that tumors don't grow as fast when treated with CBD versus with no treatment, CBD is still not as effective as traditional treatments. To me, promising evidence to indicate CBD as a supportive treatment alongside traditional medicine may help in slowing tumor growth seems to exist.

Stimulating a weak appetite

For animals with a poor appetite, CBD is a friend. (And no, this form of cannabis won't give your cat the munchies!) In more of a roundabout way, CBD has been known to interact with the serotonin receptors that regulate mood, anxiety, and a bit of the stress response. Suppressing the symptoms that diminish the appetite (body tension, stress-induced stomachaches, and more) creates space to inspire consumption.

Terpene profiles (see Chapter 2) can stimulate the appetite. With the strong presence of *terpenes* (plant chemicals) in cannabis, a good full-spectrum profile is a good combo to boost a weak appetite. Full- or broad-spectrum hemp extracts containing the terpenes myrcene, beta-caryophyllene, and limonene are the most supportive for stimulating appetite. Think mint, basil, pepper, and citrus as the flavor profiles associated with these terpenes. These aren't maybe the most appealing flavors for pets, so flavor is the one major difference between tinctures made for humans and those made for animals.

When you buy a new tincture for your friend, look at the certificate of authenticity (COA) for the terpenes.

Some companies are doing a better job than others catering specifically to animals, but if all you have at home is a human-specific tincture, it may be worth a shot. Just make sure to use the dosing recommendations in the later section "Starting low." Treat three times a day for a severe case and twice a day for mild symptoms.

Saying Goodbye to Seizures

Seizures are a neurological condition that affects cats and dogs far and wide. Not knowing what they're going through and wanting to help them is scary. The neuroprotective and anti-inflammatory properties of CBD provide an opportunity here.

Reducing the frequency of seizures

CBD combats seizures and relieves involuntary muscle spasms. All the clinical trials, actual human evidence, and the FDA-approved anti-seizure drug Epidiolex prove that CBD is effective in treating seizures. Can you believe it? I said "prove." A rare case in CBD, but the FDA says it's okay to make that claim. The drug is made from isolated CBD from the natural plant. In the studies, it was said to reduce patients' frequency in the trials by a whopping 54 percent. That's more than half the time!

Though seizures may be predicted if apparent triggers are there, most seizure medication is designed to be taken regularly to prevent the onset altogether. Because of the severity of these conditions, CBD has few downsides compared to alternative treatments for seizures. For pets, these downsides are tiredness or potentially diarrhea depending on the form administered.

Relieving epilepsy

Epidiolex, the seizure medication I earlier in the chapter, is indicated specifically for the treatment of seizures associated with Dravet syndrome and Lennox-Gastaut syndrome, two forms of epilepsy that are considered treatment-resistant in human patients. Dravet syndrome is also found in dogs. The success of Epidiolex is vital to understanding the tremendous potential CBD shares with our pet friends. Furthermore, clinical trials on dogs are happening as we speak to evaluate the efficacy specifically for cannabis. Early results are fantastic, with almost 90 percent of dog patients seeing a reduction in seizure activity.

SOURCING THE POINT OF ORIGIN FOR CBD AND SEIZURES

Dravet syndrome (and the like) typically claim the lives of patients at a young age and can be characterized by up to 100 seizures a day. Epidiolex was legalized under "compassionate use" considerations for these debilitating conditions; it's still being studied for other cases. But although it's focused on improving the quality of life for families in dire circumstances, it's also potentially positioned as a starting point for CBD in the drug market without overturning the history of cannabis prohibition in one fell swoop.

Similarly, in a compassionate use case CBD was tested, successfully, on a young child with a family that had nowhere else to turn, and that may have led to the creation of Epidiolex itself. That compassionate case is Charlotte Figi. Known (maybe) as the single most important person in the contemporary movement to overturn the media's perception of cannabis as the big bad wolf. Sanjay Gupta was compelled to tell the story of this young girl in 2013. Little Charlotte had her first seizure within months of being born. By 2 years old, she was on over seven different medications, and the doctors were stumped. At 2-and-a-half she was diagnosed with Dravet syndrome. By age 5, she was having over 300 grand mal seizures a week, and her development had been arrested. Charlotte's parent had heard about a child's success reducing seizures with cannabis. Cannabis was still illegal at the time. With nowhere left to turn, they tried it — and, amazingly, the seizures let up. This led to Charlotte's family connecting with the Stanley brothers, who had grown a strain of high-CBD, low-THC cannabis that had no market value. When both parties linked up, it became obvious they needed to try something together. Basically giving away the product, the Stanly brothers provided Charlotte and her family the CBD medicine Charlotte needed to go down to two to three seizures per month. This strain of cannabis created by the Stanley brothers is now lovingly called Charlotte's Web. It's also the name of their wildly successful brand, sold nationwide.

Getting Good with Dosing

Dosing is very much a matter of weight and the condition you're trying to treat. Due to their size, animals tend to need far less CBD than people do. Unless you're treating a horse, of course!

TIP

The Pet Hemp Company offers products for dogs, cats, and horses. They also share a nice dosing chart and calculator, which is an excellent place to look for any dosing recommendations. You can simply enter your purpose, the weight of your animal, and the strength of a tincture to uncover what is best for your pet: https://pethempcompany.com/pages/cbd-dosage-chart-for-dogs-cats.

Starting low

As with human dosing, the rule is to start slow and low for pets. You don't want to get ahead of the process, however eager you are to find relief for your furry friend. Pets' bodies also need time to adjust when you introduce something new.

The starting dose for mild symptoms is 0.25 milligrams of CBD per pound of pet:

Weight in pounds × 0.25 milligrams = Dose size in milligrams

For severe symptoms and chronic conditions, up it to 0.5 milligrams per pound:

Weight in pounds × 0.5 milligrams = Dose size in milligrams

The recommended dose frequency varies by condition:

>> For treating something like separation anxiety or stress from a trigger, you want to treat for an onset time 30 minutes before the trigger event. If you're using a treatment that has to process through the digestive tract, remember that those have a longer onset window of up to an hour and adjust accordingly. This would mean giving them the treat an hour and a half before the trigger event. If fireworks go off at 9:00, treat your pet at 7:30.

>> For pain, severe anxiety, and painful inflammation, three times a day at regular intervals is a great way to keep it consistently in your pet's system.

>> Seizures, epilepsy, and cancer can also fall into the category in the preceding bullet, but they likely also contain other layers of consideration, so keep an eye out for reactions (see the following section).

>> For all other uses (mild anxiety, prevention, gut health, and as a supplement), once or twice a day may be sufficient.

Watching for reactions

If your pet is taking any other medications, which interact with the liver, use all CBD treatments with a degree of caution. And please check with your vet. More and more veterinary practitioners are opening up to the idea of CBD, so many of them are well versed on how it works, and what other medications it can be taken with. Don't be shy. Ask away.

Anything out of the ordinary, other than a reduction in the symptoms you're trying to address, is worth paying attention to as a potential adverse reaction. Signs of distress can appear in all sorts of ways:

>> Vomiting, lack of appetite, and stomach issues like diarrhea

>> Fever

>> A yellowing tinge that can be noticeable most directly in the eyes

>> Excessive urination

WARNING

More severe reactions can include neurological problems, seizures, and blood clotting.

Adjusting as necessary

Three days is an appropriate amount of time to determine whether the dose needs to go up or down. Make sure to maintain consistency during those three days. If you find that the does isn't working, dose up by half and test for another three days. Lather, rinse, repeat.

If you've gone through this process for two weeks and see no noticeable adjustments, your pet may be unreactive to CBD. Or you may find that the brand you purchased just isn't the right one, or that the product has expired or doesn't actually have the advertised amount of CBD (this product market has very few legal food regulations on it these days). You may just find that your dog runs around the corner after you give them a treat and spits it out!

You know your animal best. After you see how they respond on a consistent dose, you'll know whether you need to do it more or less often. For example, if your pet seems a little drowsy, and that's unusual, you may need to dose down a bit. Cut out a quarter of your dose for three days and see whether that's effective. If you see a tummy reaction that lasts longer than three days, you may need to adjust the kind of CBD you're giving. The oil in the sublingual may not agree with their stomach. For the most part, I'd expect you to see a little pep in your pet's step with regular CBD use. Those looking for comfort during the end of life may have a bit more relaxation in their eyes.

4

Concocting Your Own CBD Products

Chapter **16**

Bringing CBD into the Kitchen

The options for leveling up your CBD consumption at home and in your kitchen are too fun to pass up. Did you know that you can create your own CBD bases and enhance well-loved recipes you already use with CBD products? The "secret ingredient," if you will, creates noticeable results that'll keep you coming back for more.

Discovering Ways to Add CBD to Your Regular Meals

CBD is a party animal ready to come through and jazz up any meal, day or night. The CBD marketplace has tons of different CBD products that allow you to get creative in the kitchen. CBD is also phenomenally, and I mean phenomenally, easy to use. CBD sublinguals in oil and alcohol-based tincture formats can be incredible additives to so many recipes.

Premade goodies like CBD chocolate bars make fun additions. You can chop, grind, or melt them for any number of treats like cookies, homemade chocolate milk, or even chocolate dipped bananas. I can't even imagine all the possibilities. (And I don't want to give you firm parameters and stifle your curiosity in the process. My suggestions are just that — suggestions. Be sure to have fun; that's the most important part.)

Other products on the marketplace include CBD hot sauces, honeys, seasonings, and olive oils. Products like these are designed specifically to enhance your cooking experience. Also, because they're so directly related to their non-CBD cousins, they're pretty self-explanatory.

Bringing CBD into your breakfast routine

In Chapter 8, I discuss the idea of habit stacking, where you work a new habit into an existing routine instead of creating a new routine around it. That way, your new habit is kind of like a Trojan horse, and you can incorporate it with minimal disruption.

Here's a perfect example of how to use the skill in your daily life. If you eat breakfast daily, take full advantage of that continuity! Consider sprinkling CBD granola on top of your yogurt parfait or overnight chia seed pudding for texture and added goodness.

If savory is your thing, you're in luck! The flavor palettes of many of the CBD oils on the marketplace (including CBD-infused olive oil) make a great complement to any of your breakfast culinary delights. Why not make sure your breakfast of choice has these added supplemental benefits?

REMEMBER

Just be sure to not cook these oils at very high temperatures; you don't want to burn the oil. As an alternative, you can add it as a topping after you cook just to be safe.

Many of the flavors in a full- or broad-spectrum CBD extract are really earthy and natural tasting. They go quite well with a French-style breakfast that has a side salad. The pairing is also ideal with anything that can benefit from some herbal garnish. You can easily change up your CBD oil by adding mint, basil, or parsley.

TIP

Here are six easy ways to incorporate CBD into morning meals:

>> **Olive oil:** A simple drizzling of CBD-based olive oil not only enhances the flavor of your scrambled eggs but also gives you all the antioxidant benefits an olive oil provides. Add a dash of CBD olive oil on top of your scrambled

eggs, with a sprinkling of mint to amp up the terpenes in your full-spectrum CBD.

>> **Hot sauce:** One of my favorite dishes is eggs cooked in a slow cooker with spicy roasted tomatoes and sausage. Nothing brings out these flavors more than a dash of hot sauce. Try spicing it up with Potli brand CBD hot sauce.

>> **Chocolate:** Some crushed CBD chocolate is an easy addition on top of your granola or oatmeal. Or maybe chocolate chip pancakes are in order. Crumble a CBD chocolate bar into the batter before you throw them on the griddle. Yum! You may even be able to find a CBD chocolate bar filled with dried blueberries that would yield a delicious trifecta like chocolate chip blueberry CBD pancakes. Triple whammy. I think the Calivolve brand does beautiful chocolates with a host of other beneficial ingredients beyond just the CBD. Grön chocolates also offer myriad options that can be quite fun for sweet treats and additives.

>> **Smoothie ingredients:** Smoothies also seem like a no-brainer. Just add a dose of your CBD oil as you're making your smoothie and blend it in with the other flavors. I'd even go so far as to add half a cup of hemp hearts for added protein, a fuller body, and proper endocannabinoid hemp supplementation. Smoothies are a great place for CBD honey (see the later bullet), which is a breeze to incorporate. You may even consider adding a CBD drink powder to your smoothie. That all depends on the flavor, of course, but they can be great alternatives to an oil or a honey.

>> **Nut butters:** Some CBD nut butters are coming to market that may be a great option. Take a look at Groovy Butter brand for some options and ideas. You can also DIY your own cannabutters and CBD nut butters by mixing your CBD oil directly into a standard nut butter or a butter. Stir some into your oatmeal for a breakfast treat.

>> **Honey:** So many people already add honey to their morning tea, coffee, and even cereals. A plethora of really cool CBD honeys are available on the market. They taste delicious and have the additional healing properties of a honey.

If you find that you need or want to make your own CBD honey, you're not alone! It's become a surprisingly popular endeavor. I suggest using a really high concentration CBD oil so that you're not diluting the consistency or the flavor of the honey too much by adding a higher volume of base oil.

Elevating evening meals with CBD

Breakfast (see the preceding section) isn't the only enhanceable meal option. Think about all the ways that some form of oil appears in the preparation, cooking, and presentation of a nice evening meal. Many people use it for garnish or prep; as I note in the preceding section, olive oil is typically best left unheated in order to preserve the natural antioxidant properties. And that's just one ingredient.

TIP

Here are eight easy ways to incorporate CBD into evening meals:

>> **Salad dressing:** Make your salad dressing as you normally would and add a dash of CBD oil. Generally, the servings of CBD oil are so small that it's not going to throw off the concentration of all the other ingredients in your salad dressing. You can also start your dressing with CBD olive oil; head to Chapter 11 for that recipe.

>> **Macaroni and cheese:** Infuse your butter or even your milk with CBD flower and make a delectable mac and cheese. The process of infusing is so simple. To create the perfect consistency and combination of ingredients, heat your butter a little earlier and add some cannabis flower to it. This way, you can infuse all the good flavor and supplemental benefits.

>> **Salsas:** Jazz up any of your salsas with a dash of CBD oil and a variety of herbs to complement the flavors. Like with salad dressings, the volume of CBD isn't going to affect the flavor balance of the salsa. Chopped fresh hemp leaves (if you can get your hands on them) are an awesome addition as well; think of them like cilantro or another herb. Hemp leaves aren't just beneficial from a fiber standpoint; they're also a great way to really bring that full-spectrum aspect home.

>> **Sauce:** Salsas and sauces carry some similar properties, so adding CBD extract to your sauce can be a perfect enhancement. Depending on the base of your salsa, however, your additive of choice may be different. You may want to consider an alcohol tincture extract rather than an oil if your sauce is water based because oil and water don't mix. But if the sauce is oil based or has a fatty texture, CBD oil does just fine.

>> **Sautéed veggies:** Rather than sautéing veggies in CBD oil (which requires heating the oil), I prefer steaming them and adding the oil afterward for that sautéed feeling. Simply drizzle the olive oil (or any other oil you choose) with a dash of CBD oil for an added boost.

>> **Lasagnas:** Because most pastas come from the Italian persuasion, an oil, such as olive, is going to be the most desirable option here. Make sure to add it at the right point in your cooking. Factor in the concentration and dose based on how many servings you're preparing. If you are planning on making the CBD addition part of your sauce for the lasagna, see the sauce section above, and remember that cooking temperatures above 350 degrees will compromise the CBD, so if you need to lower the cooking temperature and cook longer, go ahead. Another option would be to drizzle a finishing oil with CBD across the top of the lasagna when it is finished cooking.

>> **Deviled eggs:** Now, I wouldn't say deviled eggs are necessarily my specialty. But my mother used to call me to the kitchen to make them because she liked my combination of mustard and spicy additives. I recommend a CBD hot sauce here (see the preceding section), but if that's not your thing, you've got options. Think about using your proper dose of CBD oil in your egg yolk mixture. I think a little dash of cayenne and paprika really helps bring out the flavors.

TIP

Add black peppercorns. Cracked black pepper has a lot of the terpenes found in cannabis and enhances the experience.

>> **Cakes:** Hey, dessert is part of the evening meal, too! One of my favorite treats is a chocolate cake drizzled with lemon-flavored CBD oil. The droolworthy goodness is a whole different level of awesome.

Satisfying Your Sweet Tooth

This section is where I start to dive into the age-old tradition of cannabis treats. CBD cookies may not be the specialty your grandmother giggled about over tea with her friends when you weren't looking, but that doesn't mean they aren't just as good.

REMEMBER

Moderation is king here. The sweets may be easy to whip up, but they're even easier to knock back. Having just one brownie or gummy may be a challenge. I urge you to dose accordingly based on what you think your treat serving size will be. When you have the luxury of making your sweets at home, consider whether you're going to eat one gummy or a handful to get your dose. Because if you make them right, you may just want that handful.

Fashioning DIY CBD gummies

CBD gummies are one of the most desirable treats on the marketplace. Who doesn't like to consume tiny, yummy snacks? Here's a quick recipe you can do at home in an all-natural, healthy way. I prefer these bad boys to most of what's available in the marketplace because they have healthy ingredients. They don't rely on corn syrup, which is the number one or two ingredient in most gummies on the market, and even more exciting is that you get to choose your flavor.

These gummies are made with CBD concentrate, and the recipe yields approximately 50 gummies, 3 gummies per serving for 1 full dose of CBD. From start to finish, you can expect them to take about 45 minutes (including chilling time), though consider allowing yourself an hour as you get accustomed to the process. As soon as you find your sweet spot with these gummies, you'll be whipping out these babies in no time flat.

1. **Put 1½ cups of water or juice in a small saucepan and evenly sprinkle ½ cup of unflavored gelatin over the liquid without stirring; allow it to stand for two minutes.**

2. **Heat the mixture over medium to low heat, stirring as it heats up to help it liquefy, until it reaches 165 degrees Fahrenheit.**

   Using a candy thermometer is crucial at this point. This tool helps you be assured of the consistency and produce a good end result.

3. **Turn off the heat and pour 1½ cups of fruit puree into the liquid gelatin; whisk well.**

   Note: Don't use pineapple, ginger, kiwi, guava, or figs in your puree, as they will break down the gelatin.

4. **Add 12 doses of full-spectrum high-powered CBD distillate; whisk well to make sure the ingredients are well combined.**

5. **Pour the mixture into a large glass baking dish.**

   Alternately, you can use a pipette to fill a silicone gummy mold with the mixture.

6. **Chill the dish/mold in the fridge for 30 minutes.**

Voilà! Done. You can store your gummies in an airtight container in the refrigerator for seven days or in the freezer for up to three months.

Swapping in cannabutter

Cannabutter (butter infused with cannabis) may be one of the oldest traditions in baking with cannabis. Baked goods often require a fatty, buttery base, which makes them an easy and obvious choice for CBD infusions. Maybe it's because of the sheer ease of infusing butter with cannabis, or maybe it's because of the ease of using cannabutter in a recipe; either way, cannabutter is a good thing to know how to make.

REMEMBER

This formula and process aren't exclusive to butter. You can apply the same techniques and math to coconut oil, olive oil, ghee, or just about any other oil or fat except for margarines (because they won't go back to the same form after this process). My go-to is coconut oil because I love the versatility.

In this section, I share three common ways to make a cannabutter. Any natural butter works, but I use a grass-fed and grass-finished butter as the base because it contains no added hormones or genetically modified organisms (GMOs) for your cannabis/CBD to compete with in your system. I like the Kerrygold brand; it has fewer impurities and a higher butterfat content, which means more fats for the cannabinoids to bind to — and thus potentially a richer cannabinoid infusion.

REMEMBER

Some cannabutter methods require *decarboxylation,* or the process of activating the cannabinoids in your cannabis. I cover decarbing more deeply in the later section "Diving into decarbing."

Making cannabutter

Option one for creating your own cannabutter is to use the incredible new devices on the market that make it as easy as measuring your butter and CBD and pushing a button. My go-to device to is the Levo II, available on `www.levooil.com`. I personally share recipes using this company's device on social media because it's just so easy — no decarboxylation needed here. Other brands also have devices designed for cannabis infusions. I can't speak from experience, but several of my friends also trust the Ardent-brand infuser.

The second option is the good old-fashioned infusion device: a slow cooker. I like to use this method if I don't want to decarb the flower first. I tend to use it more for topicals, though, because the flavor is less important. I prefer the smell (over the taste) of the full plant that comes through in this longer method. Simply add your ground flower to the butter in your cooker, cover, and cook on low for three hours. If your cooker runs hot, you can add a teaspoon of water so that burns off before your butter burns. Check it often.

TIP

I generally snag my slow cookers at thrift stores. People are constantly upgrading their devices, and most of these beauties end up in the donation pile. Save that money for your good-quality cannabis flower and base butter!

The third option is the cook-top method. It's a slow and low process like the slow-cooker method, and you likely have most of the tools already; it's just the double-boiler system.

1. **Set up your double-boiler.**

   If you have a double-boiler for the stovetop, great. If not, fill a saucepan with water. Fill a heat-safe jar halfway with your butter and place it in the pan.

2. **Simmer until the butter melts and then add your ground flower to the butter.**

3. **Cook on a low simmer for three hours, adding water to the saucepan as needed to ensure it doesn't cook off.**

   Make sure the water in the pan isn't high enough to simmer over the edge and into your butter mixture.

4. **After three hours, remove from the heat.**

REMEMBER

The second and third methods require that you pour your cannabutter through a fine sieve or cheesecloth into your final container to separate the plant matter from the butter before the butter cools. You may need to do so a couple of times to make sure your butter doesn't contain particles. Store the cannabutter in an airtight jar or container in the fridge until you are ready to use it. It should be good for about a month, or in the freezer for up to six months.

A fourth method for making cannabis butter has only recently become available with the access to CBD almost nationally. Simply buy a distillate or other oil-based extract like a tincture. Measure out your butter and CBD based on the desired dose size and number. Melt the appropriate amount of butter slowly and on a low temperature; you can use any of the devices in the other methods. Then add the CBD and remove it from the heat. Stir until the extract is fully dissolved into the butter, and you're done!

TIP

Distillates like shatter, wax, rosin and similar, more-solid forms are better bets than an oil extract because the concentration of CBD is higher, so you have less interference with the additional oil and matter like you would with a sublingual oil. If you decide to use a sublingual oil, use a high-dose variety so you don't have to add as much oil to the recipe.

Calculating the CBD content in your cannabutter

When you're making a cannabutter, you need to know how much CBD is in a serving of the butter so that you can then do the math on how many milligrams of CBD are in every serving of whatever you're making.

1. **Multiply the amount of flower (in grams) you're using by 1,000 to convert the measurement to milligrams.**

   For example, say you're working with five grams of flower with 23 percent CBD. Your conversion to milligrams looks like this:

   5 grams of flower × 1,000 = 5,000 milligrams of flower

2. **Multiply the percentage of CBD in the flower by the weight of the flower in milligrams (the result from Step 1).**

   This step will give you a good estimate of the total number of milligrams in the entire batch. You should be able to find the percentage of CBD (and other cannabinoids) on the label of your flower. In this example,

   5,000 milligrams × 0.23 = 1,150 milligrams CBD

3. **Divide the amount of CBD (the result from Step 2) by the amount of butter in tablespoons to determine the amount of CBD per tablespoon of butter.**

   This approach gives you a framework to use if you're planning on using your cannabutter for various things. If you add the CBD from this example to 1 cup of butter (16 tablespoons), the math looks like this:

   1,150 milligrams CBD ÷ 16 tablespoons = 71.875 milligrams of CBD/tablespoon

TECHNICAL STUFF

Alternately, you can do a specific batch with the correct amount of butter for the base and add only as much flower as you need to reach the appropriate dose. I tend to prefer the first method because I like to use cannabutter in various ways, and whipping up a new batch of butter every time I'm making something new is too time consuming.

Note: This is a hypothetical example. In this instance, I'd personally want less CBD per dose, so I'd either increase the amount of butter (if I were going to use it all up in a month) or decrease the amount of flower I used in the butter.

REMEMBER

If you don't know the percentage of CBD in your flower and decide to try the cannabutter anyway, go low and slow. You used to be able to guesstimate average cannabinoid content in just any old flower by checking a few characteristics, but the industry has gotten so vast that this technique just isn't possible anymore. Start with a small batch so you don't end up wasting it.

BROWNIE MARY

Have you heard of the famous (sometimes infamous) Brownie Mary? You can find her full story on the internet, but she's well known in the context of San Francisco cannabis culture for offering cannabis brownies to aid ailing and terminal AIDS and HIV patients. Her baked goods were a remedy for all the nasty side effects of various medications and diseases. What a great and heartwarming story that is!

TIP

In any recipe that requires butter, you can substitute cannabutter. Cookies, brownies, magic bars, granola bars, toffees, crumbles, trail mix — you name it. The same goes for anything you may want to slather butter on top of (like, say, a muffin) to make it moister and more delectable. Just remember that the more flavorful the item you're baking, the less likely you are to taste the CBD. (And if you're using an isolate-based CBD butter, you won't taste a thing outside the traditional recipe.)

Selecting a Quality Base Oil

The bases (that is, the fatty ingredients that bond with the CBD) are the first step in creating CBD edibles of any sort. (In Chapter 2, I talk about lipids!) These ingredients are all types of cooking oils, butters, and butter substitutes (which are largely made of oils themselves).

TIP

My favorite oil of all time for cooking and to use as a CBD carrier oil is coconut oil. You can get all sorts of beautiful coconut oils at almost any store these days. Coconut oil is amazing for breakfast sweets and for all sorts of Asian cuisines, though I often find it a little harder to cook with when I'm just making scrambled eggs or something a little bit more savory. Coconut oil does tend to have a little bit of sweetness to it, and inevitably you taste the coconut flavor.

If you're looking for a more refined version of coconut oil, you can get *medium-chain triglyceride* oil (MCT). This oil is great because it always stays in oil format, whereas coconut oil is temperature sensitive and hardens in cooler and more temperate climates. The further refinement really eliminates that coconutty flavor from MCT.

Other oils like sesame oil, olive oil, or vegetable oil are pretty much interchangeable, so choose what suits you and consider your cooking style. Knowing the healthiest version of your preferred snack is a really good start to making the right selection.

TIP

For butter, I'm partial to Kerrygold grass-fed cow's butter because it has a great flavor. It's said to be much healthier in the digestive system than grain-fed cow's butter. When that isn't an option, I almost always go for organic butter, with no added hormones. When I can avoid mystery additives, that's a priority.

The quality of a base oil is debatable. Some people prefer completely unrefined options. Some people prefer virgin, and some people have no preference. I tend toward the less refined versions because I like the idea of a whole plant extract. The process of refining removes some of the active chemicals and also requires a degree of heat, which can kill off valuable antioxidants. One of my favorite brands for coconut oils is Dr Bronner's because its sourcing, packaging, and distribution process gives back as much as it takes. Any other oils I think are best organic; otherwise, you run the risk of pesticide contamination.

All in all, when it comes to oils, be discerning. You're taking CBD to heal your body. Anything that's a simple full-spectrum CBD in a natural (edible) oil without any other additive ingredients is a must-have when you're looking to cook with CBD.

Getting Familiar with Special Techniques

Everybody cooks differently. For many, cooking isn't mere meal preparation; it's an experience. Cooking with CBD is pretty much the same as cooking without it, but you should keep in mind a few techniques to ensure the best results.

Investing in quality cookware

Okay, okay, cookware isn't exactly a technique. But good technique goes only so far if you have lousy equipment.

The most important piece here is making sure that whatever you're cooking with isn't contaminating your food. Ultimately, I'd steer away from nonstick coated pans. Utensils can scrape the coating off the pan during the cooking process, and those tiny specks can end up in your food.

Stainless steel and cast iron can handle all sorts of heat variations on a stovetop and in an oven. If you're baking, consider silicone pans, or at least silicone or paper cups to line your baking dishes (especially if those dishes are nonstick). If possible, choose a glass baking dish, and remember to coat the sides and bottom with cooking oil or butter to prevent sticking.

Turning down the heat

The most important technique you need to consider when cooking with CBD is *managing your heat*. Too much heat isn't a good thing. It can not only oxidize (compromise) the oil unnecessarily but also ultimately kill off the beneficial properties of the CBD before you even get to consume it.

Regulate your heat. Whenever possible, stay below 350 degrees Fahrenheit at minimum; if you can, staying below 250 degrees is even better.

Diving into decarbing

When you're cooking with cannabis flower, *decarboxylation*, or *decarbing*, is a mandatory step. Decarbing activates the cannabinoid molecules so that you get your intended effect. It's also quite simple after you've done it.

When you're decarbing flower on its own, you must use an oven. Remember, ovens are finicky, and every oven is different. They're not all the same temperature continuously. An oven can fluctuate by as much as 20 degrees, so this whole process requires that you keep an eye on cannabis flower.

TIP

If you think you may do decarbing often, invest in an oven thermometer. It will save you time, energy, and potentially stress.

The tools you need for decarbing are a metal baking tray or a glass dish (I love Pyrex because it is so durable) and aluminum foil or parchment paper.

When you have your supplies, follow these steps:

1. **Place the oven rack in the middle position and preheat your oven to 225 degrees Fahrenheit.**

   Ovens are hotter at the top and cooler at the bottom. Placing your rack in the middle ensures that you're decarboxylating at the ideal temperature.

2. **As your oven is preheating, grind your flower by using a traditional cannabis grinder or a food processor.**

   I don't recommend a blender for this process because they're not really designed to deal with the level of stickiness that comes with this process. Make sure that your ground flower is at a granular size, similar to that of rice.

3. **Cover your baking tray in foil or parchment paper.**

   This layer is specifically to help remediate the intensity of the heat associated with the metal of the tray. But to be safe, use it with glass too. It makes clean up so much easier.

4. **Spread the cannabis flower across the covered tray and bake for 45 minutes.**

   Like I said, keep your eye on it! If the temperature of the oven fluctuates, you run the risk of burning your flower, which doesn't taste very good. No matter how strong the other ingredients in your recipe may be, the scorched taste will shine through.

SPRINKLING IN CBD ISOLATE

Although sprinkling in CBD isolate is completely possible, I'm not sure it's a popular route or one that I'd really recommend. That said, I'm happy to tell you about it anyway because some people do prefer just the isolated components of CBD without any of the full-spectrum or broad-spectrum aspects of the flower.

If you decide to try it, I suggest making sure that the other ingredients in your recipe are complementary to cannabis. That way, you're tapped into the broader-spectrum possibilities. For instance, sprinkling CBD isolate into a chocolate chip cookie recipe isn't going to be as holistically fulfilling or supplemental as using a full-spectrum CBD cannabutter.

Otherwise, this technique really is as simple as sprinkling your isolate into a recipe. The reality is the oil-based constitution of the CBD and the concentration of CBD in an isolate is high enough that it likely won't impact your recipe much.

CBD isolate is still an oil-based ingredient, so adding it to anything that's water-based and doesn't have an oil component is going to cause separation. Think about adding vinegar to oil when you're making a salad dressing. The vinegar doesn't have any lipid base, so it doesn't mix with the oil. When you shake it up, it suspends, but it doesn't mix. CBD isolate will do the same. Don't add it to a glass of water with lemon and expect it to do anything other than float on top. Add your isolate to another oil ingredient in the process of your cooking for the most cohesive results.

5. **Remove the baking sheet from the oven and let it cool.**

    The flower should be lightly toasted and a bit browner than it was before you put it in. After about 30 minutes your product should be cool enough for use or storage.

If you plan to store it, make sure to put it in an airtight container. If you plan to keep it around for a long time, put that container in the freezer. It can last for quite a long time, but remember, fresher is better.

TIP

If you're making a CBD butter or oil, you can achieve the same results with a slow cooker, as I describe in Chapter 4.

Chapter **17**

Testing Out Recipes at Home

CBD can make a great addition for anything from beverages to dinner. Anytime you can craft a recipe that supports your supplemental needs, you're doing your body a service. The diversity of CBD products on the market gives you lots of options, whether you choose to add a form of CBD to an existing recipe or craft a recipe around your favorite form.

For this chapter, I've asked a few friends in the cannabis industry and friends who love to cook to share some of their favorite beverages/cocktails and food items.

Some of these recipes were provided by professionals in their fields, and some recipes have been presented with metric measurements because they are more precise. I recommend that you consider purchasing an inexpensive food scale with a metric option if you want to do it as the professionals do it. If that sounds like too much, you can easily look up the closest conversion online. Easy breezy!

Mixing up CBD Beverages

You can add CBD to almost any beverage. The options are endless, so in this section, my friends and I provide a glimpse into just a few of the opportunities. Then, if you want to get creative on your own, add CBD to some of your other beverages, being careful to ensure the flavors are complementary.

TIP

You can add an oil-based tincture to the top of any beverage. It will not mix, but rather float on top. Be careful not to use ice or plastic in the beverage, as the oil will bind to the surface of the plastic or ice and you will miss some of those benefits.

CBD Chamomile Lemonade

by Amiah Taylor

PREP TIME: 5 MIN, PLUS CHILLING TIME | YIELD: 1 SERVING

INGREDIENTS

8 ounces water

1 CBD-infused tea sachet, such as Hemp Division CHILL

1 tablespoon raw honey, such as Breitsamer's Mountain Flower Raw Honey or Beechworth's Raw Honey with Honeycomb

2 ounces freshly squeezed lemon juice

DIRECTIONS

1 Heat 8 ounces of water.

2 Steep for the allotted time. Squeeze the tea sachet to get all the CBD goodness before discarding it.

3 Add the honey and lemon.

4 Stir to combine.

5 Chill in the refrigerator, or pour over ice for a quicker chill time.

Tonic for Reproductive Health

by Kristi Blustein, Founder of KHUS + KHUS Modern Herbal Infusion

PREP TIME: 10 MIN, PLUS INFUSING TIME | **YIELD: 2 8-OUNCE CUPS**

INGREDIENTS

8 grams shatavari root

5 grams wild yam root

5 grams dong quai root

2 grams licorice root

6 grams maca root

2 grams gingerroot

20 milligrams or two full droppers premium CBD

DIRECTIONS

1 Combine the herbs and 2 cups of water in a pot.

2 Bring the mixture to a boil and continue boiling, partly covered, until it's reduced by 3 cups.

3 Turn off the heat and allow the infusion to cool.

4 Strain the mixture and drink up to 1 cup three times a day for maximum results.

NOTE: This delicious tea is really grounding and invigorating at the same time.

TIP: I know these ingredients sound "out there." They did to me when I first started working with them and similar plants. You can literally go to Amazon to find them all! And for those of you with an awesome co-op food store or a natural food store nearby, you can likely find many of them there. I would always start with local options first!

TIP: You can add honey or coconut sugar to the final product for taste.

CBD Vanilla Italian Soda

by Amiah Taylor

PREP TIME: 3 MIN	YIELD: 1 SERVING

INGREDIENTS

8 ounces club soda or seltzer water, chilled

2 tablespoons sugar-free vanilla syrup, such as Torani

1 dropper CBD extract, such as Grön CBD's broad-spectrum

DIRECTIONS

1 Fill a glass with the club soda or seltzer water. The bubblier, the better.

2 Add the vanilla syrup and stir to combine.

3 Add the CBD extract and stir to combine.

Tahini Turmeric Latte

by Elise Museles (elisemuseles.com) + TONIC CBD (tonicvibes.com)

INGREDIENTS

1 cup plant-based mylk

1 tablespoon grated fresh turmeric, or 1 teaspoon dried

1 heaping grated teaspoon fresh ginger

½ teaspoon cinnamon, plus more for dusting

Pinch of fresh black pepper

1 tablespoon tahini

1 Medjool date, pitted

1 dose CBD oil, such as OG TONIC CBD

DIRECTIONS

1 Gently heat the plant-based mylk, turmeric, ginger, cinnamon, and black pepper in a pot until hot. Reduce to a simmer and then add the tahini and stir until well combined.

2 Remove the pot from the heat and pour the contents into a blender. Add the date and blend for about 45 seconds until smooth. Please note hot liquids in the blender can be explosive; make sure to put a towel on top of the lid and hold that baby down to prevent a mess.

3 Pour the mixture into your favorite mug. Dust with the cinnamon and add the CBD.

4 Give the mug a quick stir and enjoy your immune-boosting latte with a side of chill!

NOTE: Your turmeric latte just got a significant upgrade! This recipe is filled with anti-inflammatory spices (turmeric, ginger, and cinnamon) for immune-boosting benefits. If you use a CBD such as the OG TONIC oil, which contains ashwagandha and black seed oil, you're also getting stress-relieving ingredients to make it genuinely next level. Being in a calm state helps amp up your body's ability to fight off toxins and makes you less susceptible to getting sick. The black pepper helps with the bioavailability of the CBD, and the addition of creamy tahini helps with the absorption of the fat-soluble nutrients (and happens to taste ridiculously delicious, too)!

TIP: Use a blender with a variety of speeds. Hot liquids always need to be started at the lowest possible speed to keep the liquid from exploding out the top.

Dirty Mylk

by Blair Lauren Brown

PREP TIME: 5 MIN	YIELD: 1 SERVING

INGREDIENTS

½ tablespoon MUD\WTR coffee alternative

½ tablespoon Verté cacao

½ tablespoon coconut oil or MCT oil

3 to 4 ounces unsweetened nut mylk

1 serving CBD honey, such as Potli brand

DIRECTIONS

1 Heat the nut mylk and 3 to 4 ounces of water on a low heat.

2 Add the remaining ingredients.

3 Whisk/froth until combined.

4 Consume immediately.

NOTE: I'm sharing this coffee alternative with a touch of caffeine and the ritual element a morning pick-me-up affords. This recipe is also a healthy blast of the energy you need to feed your brain and body. Coconut oil, nut mylk, and honey are fat and sugar to provide your body with a few hours of added energy.

TIP: Natural sweeteners are better than a processed sugar because they contain nutrients and antioxidants. I use Potli honey because it has full-spectrum CBD in it with really good flavor, but I also find that I don't need the CBD for the nerves so much as I want it for the supplemental bene-fits. If CBD honey isn't an option for you, add your natural sweetener of choice and one dose of MCT-based full-spectrum CBD oil.

TIP: The natural theobromine and anandamide (happiness and energy-inducing compounds) in cacao break down over time, so make this drink fresh daily like a morning coffee ritual.

TIP: Cashew or macadamia nut mylk is best because these have a fatty, smooth texture that doesn't separate like almonds. Oat or coconut mylks work, but I find the coconut to be too sweet. Animal milks bind to the beneficial compounds in the plant products and prevent the body from absorbing them, so avoid those milks in this mixture.

Bulletproof Chai with CBD

by Layla Marvin

PREP TIME: 5 MIN	YIELD: 1 SERVING

INGREDIENTS

1 chai teabag

1 scoop collagen powder

½ tablespoon unsalted butter

½ tablespoon Verté Elevate CBD oil

Pinch of your preferred sweetener

1 splash of coconut mylk or nut mylk of your choice

DIRECTIONS

1 Boil 8 ounces of water and add the chai.

2 Steep the chai for 5 to 10 minutes.

3 Put the remaining ingredients in a mug or jar.

4 Blend with an immersion blender or frother until the contents are fully mixed. If you're using a lidded jar, you can screw the lid on tight and shake to mix.

NOTE: This recipe produces a creamy, spicy, warming, and filling beverage. It's our take on a bulletproof coffee, and my 13-year-old loves it. He even makes it for himself.

Bottoms Up! Indulging in CBD Cocktails

Adding CBD to alcohol may seem counterintuitive, but this area is actually where I found some of my greatest benefits with CBD. Because I'm already a consumer of alcohol, enhancing my cocktail recipes seems only natural. I tend to prefer tequila and mezcal to anything else. In general, alcohol is a downer for the system, and it spikes blood sugar — two things I don't think anybody needs more of. But agave-based forms such as tequila are uppers.

I find alcohol to be an end-of-the-day relaxation ritual. Enhancing that relaxation with a touch of CBD means I consume less booze, and I ultimately feel better the next day. Here are a few recipes to get you started.

Cacao Mezcal Heart Opener

by Blair Lauren Brown

PREP TIME: 5 MIN	YIELD: 1 SERVING

INGREDIENTS

½ tablespoon MUD\WTR

½ tablespoon Verté cacao

1.5 ounces nut mylk of your choice (use water if you don't like nut mylks)

Honey, maple syrup, or other sweetener to taste

1.5 ounces of mezcal (I love Gem & Bolt brand for its less smoky flavor)

1 dose full-spectrum CBD oil

Cinnamon and/or cayenne for garnish

DIRECTIONS

1 Heat the MUD/WTR, cacao, and nut mylk on low in a small pot, stirring vigorously until completely dissolved.

2 Add sweetener to taste and pour the mixture into a shaker filled with ice. Shake vigorously.

3 Strain the drink into a martini glass. Add the CBD oil across the top and garnish with the cayenne and/or cinnamon.

TIP: Mezcal makes a great pairing with cacao but if you prefer something a little less smoky, tequila is a great alternative.

TIP: You can infuse the nut mylk with chai teabags as you're heating it as a substitute for the MUD\WTR. A dose of a functional mushroom tincture also works as an additive because it will contain several exciting immune-supporting mushrooms.

VARY IT! If you want to make this drink alcohol-free, do it! It's equally uplifting and delicious. Warm, without the ice step, it makes a really incredible morning beverage. Actually, it's my go-to!

Citrus Sauvignon Spritzer

by Jewel Zimmer, Founder of Juna — www.juna-world.com

PREP TIME: 2 MIN	YIELD: 1 SERVING

INGREDIENTS

3 to 4 ounces Sauvignon Blanc, chilled

2 ounces club soda

1 ounce lemonade

1 dropper Juna Balance sublingual CBD

2 to 3 grapefruit or orange slices to taste

DIRECTIONS

1 Combine the wine, soda, and lemonade directly in a wine glass.

2 Garnish with the Juna Balance and citrus slices.

TIP: Sophisticated and deceptively simple, this CBD, citrus, and white wine spritz is the perfect pairing with corn- or fish-based meals and a balmy breeze.

CBD Old-Fashioned

by Jada Cash, Half Day CBD Brand

PREP TIME: 5 MIN	YIELD: 1 SERVING

INGREDIENTS

2 ounces bourbon or rye whiskey

1 teaspoon cherry syrup

3 dashes bitters

17 to 34 milligrams (½ to 1 full dropper) Half Day CBD Oil

2 to 3 Luxurado maraschino cherries for garnish

Orange peel for garnish

DIRECTIONS

1 In a rocks glass, mix the bourbon, cherry syrup, bitters, and CBD oil until combined.

2 Add a generous amount of ice.

3 Garnish with the cherries and orange peel.

NOTE: CBD oil mixes well with liquors that have complex flavor profiles that complement the terpenes in the CBD oil, including gin, tequila, and, in this cocktail, whiskey. Paired with the bitters and cherries, it's a delicious and potent way to unwind.

Raspberry Rhubarb CBD Sour

by Jamie Evans, Founder of The Herb Somm & Author of The Ultimate Guide to CBD and Cannabis Drinks: Secrets to Crafting CBD and THC Beverages At Home — www.theherbsomm.com

PREP TIME: 15 MIN	YIELD: 1 SERVING

INGREDIENTS

1¼ ounces Rhubarb Syrup, chilled (see the following recipe)

3 ounces Raspberry Tea, chilled (see the following recipe)

1 ounce fresh-squeezed lemon juice

1 egg white

CBD and/or THC tincture of your choice

Dusting of ground freeze-dried raspberries for garnish

DIRECTIONS

1 Add the Rhubarb Syrup, Raspberry Tea, lemon juice, egg white, and CBD and/or THC tincture into a cocktail shaker.

2 Dry shake (no ice!) for 20 to 25 seconds to form the finest froth.

3 Add ice and shake again to chill the ingredients.

4 Fine-strain the liquid into a chilled sour glass and garnish with the freeze-dried raspberries. Serve immediately and enjoy!

Rhubarb Syrup

2 cups chopped rhubarb

1 cup granulated sugar

1 Heat the rhubarb and 2½ cups of water in a saucepan until it reaches a boil.

2 Reduce the heat to medium-low and simmer for 20 to 25 minutes or until the water has absorbed most of the rhubarb's pink pigment. Remove from the heat.

3 Line a fine-mesh strainer with cheesecloth and place it over a bowl. Strain the rhubarb solids from the liquid and discard the cooked rhubarb.

4 Heat the rhubarb-infused water in a clean saucepan over low heat. Add the granulated sugar and stir until it has dissolved.

5 Remove the pan from the heat and let the mixture cool.

6 Funnel the liquid into an airtight swing bottle and store in the refrigerator until fully chilled.

Raspberry Tea

2 unsweetened raspberry teabags

1 Bring one cup of water to a boil in a teapot.

2 Pour the boiling water into a mug. Add the teabags and steep for 4 minutes.

3 Discard the used teabags and store the raspberry tea in the refrigerator until it's fully chilled.

NOTE: *Swing bottles* are popular for homemade syrups, liqueurs, and so on. Feel free to use another sealable bottle. I like swing bottles because they are easy to pour from.

Poplar Minted CBD Marg

by Blair Lauren Brown

PREP TIME: 5 MIN	YIELD: 1 SERVING

INGREDIENTS

2 ounces mezcal

1 ounce fresh lime juice

¾ ounce agave syrup

4 mint leaves, plus more for garnish

1 dose Verté Pour Le Sport Sublingual CBD Oil

DIRECTIONS

1 In a shaker full of ice, shake all the ingredients except the CBD oil until combined.

2 Add a generous amount of ice to a glass. Strain the mixture into the glass and garnish with the CBD oil and mint leaves.

NOTE: The earthy flavor profile of a bold CBD mixes well with the forward flavor of a reposado or añejo tequila. I like to use a CBD oil as a float on top because it coats your lips on every sip. A CBD full of limonene terpenes or a blend that includes citrus flavor profiles really brings out the margarita experience.

TIP: If you have another full-spectrum CBD oil with no flavor, that's a great option.

TIP: Don't use a plastic cup. The oil binds to the sides of the cup, and you lose lots of valuable CBD.

Aplos Margarita Mocktail

by Jessica Manley, Co-Founder of Aplos

PREP TIME: 5 MIN | YIELD: 1 SERVING

INGREDIENTS

2 ounces of Aplos CBD

½ ounce fresh lime juice

1 tablespoon agave nectar

2 dashes orange flower water (optional)

DIRECTIONS

1 Add all the ingredients with ice to a cocktail shaker.

2 Run a lime wedge around the outside of the rim of the glass, then roll the rim in salt.

3 Shake and strain over fresh cubes of ice into a tumbler.

4 With a peeler, cut an orange twist. Express the oils into the cocktail.

5 Garnish with a lime wheel.

NOTE: CBD in the perfect dose in an herbal beverage, made possible by Aplos brand. It creates the feeling, the ritual, and the appeal of a cocktail without the alcohol.

Cooking with CBD

Whether you're pairing it with food or integrating it into a recipe, CBD offers you the same benefits as consuming an off-the-shelf product. Integrating hemp-based proteins, another consumable hemp byproduct, can actually support your endocannabinoid system on a deeper level. The following recipes are a starting point for the variety of ways you can incorporate CBD into your food.

Skillet Sweet Potato Cornbread

by Amiah Taylor (adapted from ontysplate.com)

PREP TIME: 10 MIN	COOK TIME: 22 MIN	YIELD: 10 SERVINGS

INGREDIENTS

1¼ cups white cornmeal

1 cup self-rising flour

⅛ cup light brown sugar

½ teaspoon baking powder

½ teaspoon baking soda

¼ teaspoon nutmeg

¼ teaspoon cinnamon

½ teaspoon salt

1 cup organic nut mylk

1 cup mashed sweet potato

2 eggs, lightly beaten

½ cup butter, melted, plus more for greasing

1¼ teaspoons vanilla extract

10 doses of CBD honey, such as Cannahoney

DIRECTIONS

1 Preheat the oven to 375 degrees Fahrenheit. Melt a little less than a tablespoon of butter in the microwave and then saturate a paper towel and spread the butter evenly onto a cast-iron skillet.

2 Combine the dry ingredients one by one in a large bowl.

3 Place the nut mylk in a separate bowl and then incorporate the sweet potato, eggs, butter, and vanilla extract. Take special care not to overmix the ingredients at this stage.

4 Combine the contents of the two bowls and whisk gently until just combined.

5 Transfer the batter into the skillet and bake for 18 minutes until it's a little brown on the top. If the top is still soft, bake for 4 more minutes.

6 Let the bread cool and then slice it. Drizzle the honey all over the slices.

TIP: If the oven hasn't reached 375 degrees by the time you have the batter mixed, refrigerate the batter until the oven is ready.

Sweet Potato, Brussels, Sardine, and Egg Hash

by Jamie Truppi, MSN, CNS, Functional Nutritionist & Edible Educator

PREP TIME: 5 MIN	COOK TIME: 16 MIN	YIELD: 2 SERVINGS

INGREDIENTS

1 sweet potato

½ cup Brussels sprouts

2 tablespoons coconut oil

1 can (4 to 5 ounces) sardines or canned wild salmon

½ teaspoon finely chopped or ground rosemary

4 eggs

Black pepper to taste

Sea salt to taste

2 tablespoons sauerkraut

DIRECTIONS

1 Dice the sweet potato into small cubes and chop the Brussels sprouts.

2 Heat the coconut oil in a large skillet (with lid) over medium heat.

3 Add the sweet potatoes to the skillet and cook, covered, for 4 minutes or until they begin to brown. Flip them over and add the Brussels sprouts. Sauté 4 to 5 more minutes until the sprouts are brighter.

4 Meanwhile, roughly chop the sardines or drain the canned salmon. Add the fish to the veggie mixture along with the rosemary.

5 Drop the eggs one at a time on top of the veggies. Cover and allow the eggs to poach to your desired yolk firmness (about 5 to 7 minutes).

6 Season to taste with black pepper and sea salt. Garnish with the sauerkraut and enjoy!

NOTE: This simple breakfast, lunch, or dinner recipe is rife with foods that contain beneficial nutrients that support the body's endocannabinoid system (ECS; see Chapter 3) so adding CBD isn't necessary. Sweet potato supports the endocannabinoid system activity in the brain. Cruciferous vegetables such as Brussels sprouts bind to CB2 and reduce inflammation. Omega-3 fatty acids from low-mercury fish such as sardines and wild salmon support cannabinoid receptors. So does the nutrient beta-caryophyllene in rosemary and black pepper. Finally, sauerkraut is a probiotic-rich food that increases activity of CB2 receptors.

TIP: Use pasture-raised eggs; they're more beneficial and contain precursors to the body's natural cannabinoids.

VARY IT! In Step 5, you can scramble the eggs into the mixture by breaking up the yolks and then sautéing until the eggs are cooked through.

Gado Gado Salad

by Ujin Kim of Potli

PREP TIME: 15 MIN	COOK TIME: 10 MIN	YIELD: 3 SERVINGS

INGREDIENTS

7 ounces (or half of a package) tempeh or choice of protein

1 head of butter lettuce (or favorite greens)

3 medium carrots, roughly chopped

1 cup bean sprouts

2 sliced shallots

2 hard-boiled eggs

1 tablespoon Potli Awaken Apple Cider Vinegar

1 tablespoon sesame oil

½ cup peanut butter

1 tablespoon soy sauce (or coconut aminos)

1 clove of minced garlic

1 dash smoked paprika

1 tablespoon Potli Extra Vibrant Olive Oil

Salt and pepper to taste

9 wheat or rice crackers

DIRECTIONS

1 Marinate tempeh in a mixture of Potli Awaken Apple Cider Vinegar and soy sauce. Bake 350-degree oven for 10 minutes, turning midway through.

2 Clean and chop vegetables. Slightly blanch bean sprouts or carrots if desired.

3 Toss greens and protein together into a salad bowl.

4 Boil eggs for 8 minutes on medium heat.

5 Prepare the salad dressing by combining peanut butter, soy sauce, sesame oil, minced garlic, smoked paprika, and Potli Awaken Apple Cider Vinegar until smooth.

6 Dress the salad, add sliced boiled eggs, and finish off with a light wash of Potli Extra Vibrant Olive Oil. Top off with crackers and seasoning to taste.

NOTE: Gado Gado is an Indonesian staple featuring a rich variety of textures and flavors with slightly blanched and fresh vegetables dressed in a creamy peanut butter dressing.

Caramelized Figs and Whipped Yogurt

by Maria Hines, World-Renowned Michelin-Starred Chef

PREP TIME: 15 MIN	COOK TIME: 5 MIN	YIELD: 4 SERVINGS

INGREDIENTS

1 pint fresh figs

2 tablespoons sugar

½ cup heavy cream

½ cup Greek yogurt

½ cup pistachios, toasted and crushed

¼ cup CBD honey

Sea salt to taste

DIRECTIONS

1 Slice the figs in half and sprinkle with the sugar.

2 Arrange the figs on a sheet pan, cut side up, and place it under the broiler until they're caramelized, about 2 minutes.

3 In a mixing bowl, slowly whisk the yogurt and heavy cream to firm peaks.

4 Arrange the figs on a serving plate. Dollop the whipped yogurt over the figs and sprinkle with the crushed pistachios.

5 Finish by drizzling with the CBD honey and adding sea salt to taste.

NOTE: Yogurt adds the perfect creamy, tangy accent to the sweetness of the figs. I like Greek yogurt for the sweetness and acidity.

TIP: If you have a blowtorch, you can caramelize the figs quickly in Step 2 without cooking them too much.

Creating CBD Ingredients

If you're feeling up to it, sometimes making your base ingredients for a recipe is nice. The basics, from butter to olive oil and sugar to simple syrup, are required in just about everything we make.

Simple CBD Sugar

by April Pride, cannabis entrepreneur, advocate, and investor

PREP TIME: 5 MIN, PLUS 1 TO 3 DAYS OF EVAPORATING TIME	YIELD: 1 CUP

INGREDIENTS

1 cup of sugar

1 ounce alcohol-based CBD tincture

DIRECTIONS

1 Spread the sugar over a flat surface.

2 Pour the tincture over the sugar and mix well.

3 Over the next 24 to 72 hours, mix the sugar so that the alcohol evaporates evenly. When the sugar is no longer damp, it's done!

NOTE: I like having CBD-infused sugar to add to tea any time of day. A 1-ounce tincture with 300 milligrams of CBD poured over 1 cup of sugar yields 48 teaspoons of sugar with 6.25 milligrams of CBD per teaspoon.

TIP: Be sure to use an alcohol-based tincture so the alcohol can evaporate, leaving the cannabinoids infused in the sugar. Oil-based tinctures simply can't substitute. Recipes for alcohol-based cannabis and hemp tinctures are available online.

TIP: Store this sugar in a covered sugar dish clearly labeled *Contains Cannabis* so no one accidentally doses.

CBD Simple Syrup

by Blair Lauren Brown

PREP TIME: 30 MIN	YIELD: 16 1-OUNCE SERVINGS

INGREDIENTS

1 cup water

1 cup of sugar, agave, or honey

1 tablespoon vegetable glycerin

1 ounce alcohol-based CBD tincture

DIRECTIONS

1 In a small saucepan, bring the water to a low simmer on low heat.

2 Slowly add the sugar, agave, or honey, stirring as you do.

3 Cover and simmer for 20 minutes.

4 Remove the cover and stir in the vegetable glycerin for 4 to 5 minutes.

5 Remove from the heat and stir in the CBD mixture as it cools.

6 Before it is completely cooled, poor it into the final container and leave it out until it is cool.

7 Once the mixture has cooled, you can use it or cover it and place it in the refrigerator.

NOTE: A CBD-infused simple syrup is a great addition to any beverage. A 1-ounce tincture with 500 milligrams of CBD yields 16 ounces with 31.25 milligrams of CBD per ounce.

TIP: Be sure to use an alcohol-based tincture so the alcohol can evaporate in the heating process. Oil-based tinctures will create a separation in the mixture, creating uneven doses. Recipes for alcohol-based cannabis and hemp tinctures are available online.

TIP: Store this mixture in the refrigerator covered for up to 6 months, or use it all in one fabulous dinner party.

Chapter **18**

Branching out to Other CBD and Hemp Products

atti Smith said it best: "If you feel good about who you are inside, it will radiate." I think three things let people radiate around them: nourishing themselves with tasty food, which reflects on their skin; nourishing their skin; and nourishing the ones they love. In this chapter, I explore recipes for those three elements. I also have added a couple recipes that don't have CBD in them because they illustrate valuable points. One, specifically, has hemp hearts to show you that there are other great hemp ingredients to add to recipes that have benefits to support your CBD supplementation. The other is merely a recipe — just add CBD — simply to illustrate that this is possible, easy to do, and a great option too.

Treating Your Sweet Tooth: Recipes for CBD Sweets and Snacks

Although eating sweet treats while supplementing your body with CBD, which is designed to heal, may seem counterintuitive, that's not necessarily the case. My friends and I have tapped into nourishing and healthy snacks that can satisfy your sweet tooth and address your CBD needs.

Rosebud CBD Marshmallows

by Rosebud CBD

INGREDIENTS

1 teaspoon of gelatin

¾ cup sugar

½ cup corn syrup

¼ teaspoon salt

1 tablespoon vanilla extract

1 to 2 full droppers Rosebud CBD Oil

½ cup powdered sugar

DIRECTIONS

1 Stir the gelatin and ¼ cup of cold water together in the bottom of your stand mixer's bowl. Set aside.

2 Spray a deep 8-x-8-inch baking dish with cooking spray. Line the dish with parchment paper and spray that with another light coating.

3 In a small saucepan, stir together the sugar, corn syrup, salt, and ¼ cup of water. Cook on medium-high heat without stirring until the syrup reaches 240 degrees Fahrenheit, about 10 minutes.

4 Fit the mixer with the whisk attachment and turn the mixer on low. Slowly pour all the syrup in the bowl and mix until the gelatin is dissolved.

5 Turn off the mixer and add the vanilla and CBD oil. Mix on high speed until the mixture is thick, stiff, and bright, opaque white.

6 Pour the mixture into the prepared pan and spread evenly. Let sit uncovered at room temperature for at least 4 hours.

7 Sift a bit of powdered sugar onto your workspace. Use a knife to carefully lift out the marshmallows, flipping them onto the sugared surface and then slowly peeling off the parchment paper.

8 Using a long, sharp knife, make three cuts lengthwise and then across the other direction, wiping your knife with a damp towel as needed.

9 Separate the cubes and toss them in a bowl with more sifted powdered sugar until they're thoroughly coated.

TIP: Store the marshmallows in an airtight container for up to ten days.

TIP: One dropper of 350 milligram CBD makes each marshmallow contain 2 to 4 milligrams of CBD.

Groovy Chocolate–Covered Strawberries

by Rachel Weber, founder of Groovy Butter

PREP TIME: 5 MIN, PLUS CHILLING TIME	YIELD: 2 SERVINGS

INGREDIENTS

2 tablespoons Groovy Butter CBD-infused Hazelnut Cacao Butter, room temperature

4 ripe strawberries

DIRECTIONS

1 Put the hazelnut cacao butter in a bowl.

2 Submerge the strawberries in the nut butter and place them on waxed paper.

3 Refrigerate the strawberries for 3 hours until the butter firms up into a creamy chocolate shell around them.

NOTE: Each two-berry serving contains 15 milligrams of CBD.

TIP: Serve within 2 days.

TIP: You can use any organic, unprocessed, plant-based chocolate hazelnut butter and unflavored CBD oil, thoroughly and evenly mixed. If your butter is creamy rather than drizzly, warm it up in a saucepan on low for a few moments.

VARY IT! For something different, swap in your fruit of choice.

Vanilla Cinnamon Bliss Balls

by Michelle Helfner, L.Ac.

| PREP TIME: 5 MIN, PLUS CHILLING TIME | YIELD: 18 BALLS |

INGREDIENTS

2 tablespoons CBD-infused coconut oil

1 cup cashews

½ cup dates, pitted

¼ cup coconut flour

1 tablespoon ghee

1 teaspoon vanilla extract

1 teaspoon cinnamon

Pinch of sea salt

DIRECTIONS

1 Combine all the ingredients in a bowl or food processor.

2 Mix well until the mixture looks like cookie dough.

3 Place large tablespoon scoops of dough onto a parchment-lined cookie sheet.

4 Chill in the fridge for 20 minutes.

NOTE: These bites are filled with protein and energy, balanced with CBD for a little relaxation. They're a great way to start the day or grab a snack!

TIP: You can skip the refrigerating time and eat these goodies right away, but I think they're better chilled.

VARY IT! After you get the hang of this process, you can mix and match ingredients for this recipe in many ways, so explore! Basically, start with a nut (almond, cashew, macadamia, peanut), add a sweetener (dates, honey), and then mix in spices and flavors, chia, sesame, quinoa puffs, coconut — whatever you want.

Lemon Chia Coconut Bliss Balls

by Michelle Helfner, L.Ac.

PREP TIME: 15 MIN, PLUS CHILLING TIME	YIELD: 18 BALLS

INGREDIENTS

Juice of 2 lemons (about 6 tablespoons)

2 tablespoons chia seeds

2 tablespoons honey

1½ cups quick oats

1 tablespoon CBD oil

1 cup shredded coconut, divided

DIRECTIONS

1 Combine all the ingredients in a bowl or food processor, reserving ½ cup of the coconut, and mix well.

2 Let the mixture sit for 5 to 10 minutes.

3 Moisten your hands and roll the mixture into balls.

4 Coat the balls with the remaining coconut.

5 Chill in the fridge for 30 minutes.

TIP: You can use ½ tablespoon of CBD oil to adjust for strength.

VARY IT! Head to the Vanilla Cinnamon Bliss Balls recipe in this chapter for some basic guidelines on creating your own takes on this recipe.

Cacao Chia Bliss Balls

by Michelle Helfner, L.Ac.

PREP TIME: 5 MIN, PLUS CHILLING TIME	YIELD: 18 BALLS

INGREDIENTS

1 cup dates, pitted

6 tablespoons chia seeds

1 tablespoon CBD oil

¼ cup almonds or crunchy peanut butter

3 tablespoons cacao powder

DIRECTIONS

1 Mix all the ingredients well in a bowl or food processor until sticky. If your dates are dry, add 1 teaspoon of water at a time.

2 Roll the mixture into 1-inch balls and place on parchment paper.

3 Chill in the fridge for 30 minutes.

TIP: You can roll the balls in sesame seeds or additional chia seeds in Step 2 as a topping if desired.

VARY IT! Head to the Vanilla Cinnamon Bliss Balls recipe in this chapter for some basic guidelines on creating your own takes on this recipe.

Nirvana Truffles

by Victorine Deych

INGREDIENTS

2 ripe medium organic avocados

2 bars or 2 cups Lily's dark chocolate chips

1 teaspoon vanilla

2 teaspoons coconut sugar

1 cup organic cacao powder

1 teaspoon full-spectrum CBD

1 drop limonene terpene

1 drop myrcene

1 cup shredded coconut

Zest of 1 medium organic orange

DIRECTIONS

1 Peel and pit the avocados and process in a food processor until smooth.

2 Heat the chocolate in a small pot over medium heat until melted.

3 Combine the avocado, the melted chocolate, the vanilla, the coconut sugar, the cacao powder, the CBD, the limonene, and the myrcene in a food processor.

4 When the ingredients are well mixed, add the orange zest and give the mixture one final stir.

5 With your hands or a tablespoon, scoop out the mixture and roll it into about 1-inch balls. Roll the balls in the shredded coconut and place them on a cookie sheet.

6 Chill the rolled truffles in the refrigerator until they harden.

TIP: Get your CBD and terpenes (such as the limonene and myrcene in this recipe) from an organic and reputable source. You can find terpenes from Dusted Terpenes. You can also substitute with a sprinkling of grated lemon rind.

Protein-Packed Power Cookie

by Blair Lauren Brown

PREP TIME: 15 MIN, PLUS CHILLING TIME	COOK TIME: 10–12 MIN	YIELD: 20 COOKIES

INGREDIENTS

2 sticks organic, grass-fed/finished butter

½ cup monk or coconut sugar

1 cup light brown sugar, packed

2 large eggs

1 tablespoon vanilla extract

1 teaspoon baking soda

½ teaspoon sea salt

1½ cups flour

2 cups chocolate chips

1½ cups organic hemp hearts

1 cup nuts (optional)

DIRECTIONS

1 Mix the butter and sugars until smooth. Add the eggs and vanilla and mix again.

2 Add the baking soda and salt, dispersing them as evenly as possible. Slowly add flour, mixing until it's fully incorporated. Mix in the remaining ingredients.

3 Refrigerate the dough until it's solid, about 20 to 25 minutes.

4 Preheat the oven to 375 degrees Fahrenheit.

5 When the oven is 5 minutes away from being preheated, remove the dough from the fridge and form mounded balls on an ungreased cookie sheet. Space the balls out 1 to 1.5 inches apart for room to spread out as they cook. About half of the dough will remain. You can make the second batch now on another cookie sheet or store it in the fridge for later.

6 Place in the oven immediately and bake for 10 to 12 minutes for chewy cookies or 12-to 15 minutes for crispy cookies.

NOTE: This recipe doesn't contain CBD. It contains hemp hearts, a vital addition to your food nutrients to support your endocannabinoid system (see Chapter 3). It's full of healthy fats and all the hemp protein and antioxidants needed to give you a bit of energy and support all that CBD intake you're getting elsewhere!

TIP: Ingredients from organic and natural sources are the fullest in natural and vital minerals.

Treating Your Body: Recipes for CBD Body Care and Skincare

Making CBD skincare really lets my heart sing. As a formulator in the space, I cut my teeth with a line of CBD-focused skincare products. CBD has so many skin benefits beyond just inflammation. Destressing the skin not only makes you feel good but also makes you look good.

Glowing CBD Face Mask

by Bridgetta Harden, Co-Founder of NFZD Beauty

PREP TIME: 5 MIN	YIELD: 1 USE

INGREDIENTS

1 tablespoon organic aloe vera gel

1 teaspoon of organic honey, such as manuka honey

½ dropper NFZD Beauty Illuminate and Hydrate CBD Face Oil or your favorite CBD oil

DIRECTIONS

1 Combine all the ingredients in a glass bowl.

2 Apply the mixture to a clean face with your fingers or a mask wand.

3 Leave the mask on for 15 to 20 minutes.

4 Rinse off the mask.

NOTE: This is the perfect face mask for combination skin. Make and use it twice weekly after cleaning your face; you should discard any leftovers each time. Get ready for glowing skin!

TIP: A mask wand is like a a makeup brush, but instead of having a bristled end, it's a silicone spatula of sorts.

Skin Perfecting, Smoothing, and Hydrating Omega Mask

by Carla Butts, Master Esthetician/Founder, Light + Space Skin

PREP TIME: 5 MIN	YIELD: 1 MASK

INGREDIENTS

2 tablespoons raw organic honey, such as manuka honey

1 tablespoon (3 pumps/pipettes) hyaluronic acid serum or any hydrating serum

1 tablespoon organic rosehip oil or jojoba oil

1 pipette Verté Essential Vital CBD Oil or CBD oil of your choice

½ tablespoon Verté Essentials Esprit de Rose or rosewater facial toner of your choice, plus more for finishing

Moisturizer for finishing

DIRECTIONS

1 Whisk the honey and the hyaluronic acid serum with a fan brush or whisk until well combined.

2 Fold in the rest of the ingredients thoroughly one at a time, adding the rosewater toner last. Whip the mixture until it achieves a very smooth consistency.

3 Use your fingertips or the fan brush you used in Step 1 to apply a generous layer all over your freshly cleaned face, neck, and upper décolletage.

4 Leave the mask on for 20 to 40 minutes — 20 for more sensitive skin, longer for heartier skins.

5 Press a warm, damp washcloth over the skin for about 1 minute to allow more absorption. Remove the remainder of the product with the washcloth, splash your skin with warm water, and then pat dry.

6 Spritz your skin with a bit more of the rosewater toner and pat into the skin. Finish with moisturizer and admire your glow-ing complexion!

NOTE: This facial mask is an all-in-one, absolute go-to for hydrating and smoothing the skin, revealing clear radiance. Its benefits include brightening, exfoliation, moisturizing, and the encouragement of healing.

NOTE: This mask is appropriate for any skin type and condition, including acne, for which it's very helpful. The ingredients combine to attract water and impart moisture deep into the skin. Rosehip is great for dry skin and uneven pigmentation, and jojoba oil is better for acne-prone skin. The honey offers substantial healing and anti-inflammatory benefits while also increasing cell turnover, and it activates gentle exfoliation. This, in combination with CBD and vital oils, generates a balanced, well-functioning barrier. You're sure to attract some good attention for your enviable glow after this one!

TIP: When you're ready to apply the mask, make sure you've pulled your hair back with a headband so your face is free. You may also want to wear a low-cut shirt because the mask covers your neck and décolletage.

Bath Bombs

by Raeven Duckett-Robinson, Co-Founder Community Gardens Inc.

PREP TIME: 20 MIN, PLUS OVERNIGHT DRYING TIME	YIELD: 6 BOMBS

INGREDIENTS

½ cup baking soda

¼ cup cream of tartar

¼ cup Epsom salt

10 drops essential oil(s) of your choice

2 teaspoons CBD infused olive oil

DIRECTIONS

1 Whisk the dry ingredients in a large bowl.

2 In a separate, smaller bowl, combine the olive oil, essential oils, and ½ teaspoon of water and mix them with a spoon.

3 Add your wet ingredients to your dry ingredients as slowly as possible (to prevent bubbling) while whisking. The consistency of your mixture should feel like damp sand. If it doesn't, slowly add 1 more teaspoon of water.

4 Pack the mixture tightly into silicone bath bomb molds and let dry for 24 hours.

5 Carefully remove the bath bombs from the molds and allow them to air dry undisturbed for another 24 hours.

TIP: Here are some essential oil suggestions:

Lavender and rosemary: Great for relieving insomnia

Peppermint: Great for sore muscles

Orange, lemon, and ylang ylang: Improves mood and state of being

Pine, cedar, and juniper: Great for cramps and arthritis

TIP: You can use round or square silicone molds made for either bath bombs or large ice cubes.

Spa-Style Bath Soak for Pain and Muscle Recovery

by Blair Lauren Brown, for www.mypersonalplants.com

PREP TIME: 20 MIN	YIELD: 1 SOAK

INGREDIENTS

150 milligrams CBD suspended in oil

10 drops chai essential oil blend

1 teaspoon arnica oil (suspended in sunflower oil, or plain extract will work)

1½ cups Epsom salt, divided

1 tablespoon baking soda

½ cup pink Himalayan salt

1 tablespoon clove

1 tablespoon ginger

1 tablespoon cardamom

1 cinnamon stick

1 tablespoon Alaea clay salt

DIRECTIONS

1 Combine the CBD, essential oil, and arnica oil in the bottom of a container.

2 Add 1 cup of the Epsom salt, holding the vessel flat to the tabletop surface.

3 Add the baking soda and wiggle the vessel a bit to settle. Repeat with the Himalayan salt and then again with ¼ cup of the remaining Epsom salt.

4 Combine the clove, ginger, cardamom, and cinnamon in mortar and pestle and grind. Alternately, give them a light grind in a food processor — just enough to expose the fragrant properties of the plants.

5 Add your ground botanicals to the vessel and settle until the layer reaches the side. Add the remaining Epsom salt and settle again.

6 Add the Alaea clay salt.

TIP: CBD isolate, oil, or distillate will work in this recipe. If your CBD isn't already suspended in oil, combine it with 1 tablespoon of MCT oil and the essential oil and arnica oil in Step 1 and let that dissolve into the bottom of your vessel.

TIP: Use a clear glass vessel because the layering of this soak is really beautiful to look at. For use, pour the soak into a muslin bag so the botanicals don't get stuck in the drain when you empty the bath. You can also use a fine-mesh strainer as an alternative, but you want the botanicals to continue soaking in the bath as you do for the full experience.

TIP: Making a few soaks in one sitting is a great way to be efficient with your time and then have backup on hand for when you need it. These soaks last for three months before the oil starts to degrade the botanicals.

Body Ease Polish Inflammation– Reducing Body Scrub

by Jasmine-Symonn Gates, Founder of Sincerely Bade

PREP TIME:	YIELD: 3–4 SERVINGS

INGREDIENTS

1 cup fine organic cane sugar

1 cup finely ground oatmeal

½ cup organic jojoba oil

½ cup organic sweet almond oil

¼ cup organic raw honey

2 tablespoons ground turmeric

1 teaspoon ground cinnamon

100 mg of full spectrum CBD oil

DIRECTIONS

1 In a small glass bowl, combine ¼ teaspoon of the cane sugar, the oatmeal, jojoba oil, sweet almond oil, honey, cinnamon, and turmeric until it's well blended.

2 Continue adding ¼ teaspoon of cane sugar at a time until you reach a grainy paste consistency that easily spreads across the skin. You may not need the full 1 cup.

3 Add the CBD oil and mix well.

4 Rub a bit of the mix between your hands to check consistency. It may seem oily in the bowl, but it'll absorb nicely when rubbed into the skin. If you find it's too oily, add a bit more cane sugar or ground oatmeal.

5 Store your finished product in a tightly sealed glass jar, away from water and humidity.

6 To use, gently massage a palmful of scrub onto wet skin, especially focusing on areas that may be sore or achy. Rinse after 2 to 5 minutes.

NOTE: Turmeric does have a reputation of slightly staining the skin in large quantities; however it should easily rinse off if you're using the appropriate amount of oils. Make sure your turmeric is finely ground and well-blended among the other ingredients.

TIP: I recommend keeping the scrub away from water and humidity because mold and bacteria can grow in damp environments. Try storing it tightly sealed in a glass jar in the fridge or in a bathroom cabinet. Use a spoon to dispense it, or ensure your fingers are dry before you use it.

Treating Your Pooch: Recipes for CBD Dog Food and Treats

Pets deserve a little love, too. The following recipes are specific to canine friends, but with a little modification, I'm pretty sure your cats could get in on the act.

Jade from Half Day CBD has been so kind as to share the following dosing chart to determine how much CBD to add to your recipe, depending on your dog's size and desired potency. Make sure to use a CBD brand you trust that's third-party tested for safety and potency and that has clear dosing breakdowns. Half Day CBD's Full-Spectrum 1,000 milligram formula, for example, contains 34 milligrams of CBD per 1 milliliter (one dropper).

Dog weight	Small dose	Medium dose	Large dose
Under 10 lbs	1–2 mg	3 mg	6 mg
11–25 lbs	3 mg	5 mg	10 mg
26–50 lbs	5 mg	10 mg	15 mg
51–75 lbs	10 mg	15 mg	20 mg
76 lbs and up	15 mg	20 mg	25 mg

REMEMBER

This dosing chart is still only a rough guideline because every animal is different. Look for signs that the dose is working, like a sense of calm and relaxation, or that the dose is too strong, like being overly tired or sleeping all the time.

WARNING

Make sure you aren't using artificial sweeteners, or ingredients that contain them, in your dog treats. These sweeteners, such as xylitol, can be harmful for dogs.

Pumpkin and Peanut Butter Dog Treats

by Jada Cash, Half Day CBD

PREP TIME: 10 MIN	COOK TIME: 30 MIN	YIELD: 35–40 TREATS

INGREDIENTS

One 15-ounce can pumpkin puree

2 tablespoons peanut butter free of artificial sweeteners

1 tablespoon honey

¼ teaspoon cinnamon

70 –1,200 milligrams full-spectrum or isolate CBD oil

3 cups all-purpose flour

DIRECTIONS

1 Preheat the oven to 325 degrees Fahrenheit.

2 Fit a hand or stand mixer with a whisk attachment and mix the pumpkin, peanut butter, honey, and CBD oil until very well combined. Ensure the CBD oil is evenly dispersed throughout the dough so each treat contains a consistent dose.

3 Switch to the mixer's paddle attachment and mix on low while slowly adding the flour until well combined. The dough should be smooth and not too sticky. Add a little flour (if too sticky) or water (too crumbly) as necessary.

4 Roll out the dough to about ⅛-to-¼-inch thickness. Use a small or medium cookie cutter to cut shapes out.

5 Place the cookies on a cookie sheet and bake for 30 to 40 minutes or until hard/very well done.

6 Let the treats cool thoroughly. You can store them in an airtight container for up to 2 weeks or refrigerate or freeze batches to extend their shelf life.

TIP: You can use full-spectrum or isolate CBD oil, but I recommend full-spectrum, which experts believe has a greater impact because it contains the full spectrum of cannabinoids, including trace amounts of THC. The amount of CBD oil you use will vary depending on the size of the dog and the desired potency (see the dosing chart earlier in this section for specific amounts).

TIP: Watch your oven temperature here. Cooking CBD at temperatures higher than 350 degrees can cause it to lose its beneficial properties.

TIP: You can also mix the dough by hand in Step 3.

Lucy's No Bake Anti-Inflammatory Pumpkin Dog Treats

by Alyssa Riccio, CPC &CSC, Certified Life and Spiritual Coach

PREP TIME: 10 MIN, PLUS CHILLING TIME | **YIELD: 14 TREATS**

INGREDIENTS

2 cups pumpkin puree

3 tablespoons honey

3 teaspoons turmeric

½ teaspoon cinnamon

3 tablespoons coconut oil

2 cups rolled oats

14 doses CBD oil

DIRECTIONS

1 Mix the pumpkin, honey, turmeric, cinnamon, and coconut oil in a bowl.

2 Add the oats slowly to create a cookie dough consistency. You may not need all 2 cups.

3 Roll the mixture into 14 small balls by using your hands, a melon baller, or a small ice cream scoop. Put the balls on a parchment-lined or nonstick baking sheet or plate.

4 Add a dose of CBD oil (as determined by the product label) to each ball. For doses of more than half a dropper, you may want to make a well with your finger and put the oil there to let it soak.

5 Put the balls in the refrigerator until they harden slightly, about 15 minutes.

TIP: Make sure your pumpkin puree is organic and free of sweeteners or spices.

Homemade Food for Your Fur Baby Plus CBD

by Brandelyn M. Rosenberg

PREP TIME: 5–10 MIN	COOK TIME: 20–30 MIN	YIELD: 2 TO 4 SERVINGS

INGREDIENTS

1 cup white rice, preferably organic jasmine

½ cup turkey bone broth

1 pound ground turkey

2 large carrots

1 apple

4 servings CBD tincture for serving

DIRECTIONS

1 Put the rice and 2 cups of water into a pot. Bring it to boil and then reduce the heat to low. Cover and cook until the rice has soaked up all the water.

2 Turn off the heat. Add the bone broth to the rice to moisten it and add flavor. Set aside.

3 Brown the turkey in a separate pan. Let it cool.

4 Chop the carrots and apple. Combine them with the rice and turkey.

5 Put 1 or 2 cups of the mixture (depending on the size of your dog) into your dog's bowl. Top with a dose of CBD oil.

6 Check the food's temperature with your finger to make sure it's not too hot to eat, add cold water if needed, and serve.

NOTE: I've been feeding my dog homemade dog food with all the nutrients she needs, discussing the issue with my vet as well as doing in-depth research. Because of my dog's allergies to commercial dog food brands, fatty meats, and preservatives, I stick to this recipe.

NOTE: You can store this in your fridge for up to three days, so if you need to make more in advance to save time, no problem.

TIP: If you don't want to use the apple and carrots raw, you can chop them earlier and cook them with the rice in Step 1 or with the turkey in Step 3.

TIP: If you don't have CBD in tincture form, you can substitute CBD dog treats to top off the meal.

5

The Part of Tens

Explore ten reasons to give CBD a go.

Consider ten ways that CBD can help with ailments and uncomfortable conditions.

Discover ten ways to get this good stuff into your body.

Put the icing on the cake with ten tips to help you have the best experience possible.

Chapter **19**

Ten Reasons to Try CBD

The list of reasons to use CBD is endless. The following sections list some of the more compelling ones.

You Can Use CBD Every Day

You can take CBD daily as a supplement. A supplemental dose of CBD may treat some conditions' side effects or symptoms and even potentially prevent you from experiencing these conditions at all. The compelling theories around clinical endocannabinoid deficiency (see Chapter 3) and the long history of hemp's dietary value are other concepts that support the idea of daily CBD use.

CBD Is a Plant-Based Product (Usually)

For the most part, the CBD you're likely to encounter is plant-based. It's naturally been studied from a human consumption standpoint for thousands of years.

As the industry evolves, synthesized versions of CBD will show up. Converting other chemical substances to CBD in a lab is possible (and quite easy), but as an isolated chemical, CBD is CBD. Whether its origin is synthetic or natural doesn't alter or compromise its properties.

CBD Is Safe to Use

Here's the truth: If you ask anybody in the cannabis (not just CBD/hemp) space, no one has ever fatally overdosed from using cannabis.

All of the studies and anecdotal evidence around CBD indicate that the side effects are few and far between. Most of those that may exist are only mildly relevant in the scheme of things, especially relative to what you're trying to treat.

The more serious side effects include possible contraindications with pharmaceutical or over-the-counter drugs. Some of these medications are processed through the liver, as is CBD. Check with your doctor regarding all the drugs you're taking and the spectrum of potential drug interactions between those and CBD.

CBD is also safe from the standpoint that you don't have to worry about feeling high or out of body, as I explain in the later section "CBD Doesn't Get You High."

CBD Is Easy to Ingest

CBD and its natural plant form are easy to ingest. The flower, be it the hemp or cannabis plant, has been smoked and consumed via inhalation for centuries. Later, the plant was extracted or infused for consumption. Methods of use ranged from tea to edibles long before anyone was recording potential recipes for consumption.

Now that the market has evolved and has many players, your imagination is essentially the limit. Sweets and baked goods, tinctures that taste like cookies, gums and mints, oral sprays, drinks and drink mixes — I think you get the picture.

CBD Doesn't Get You High

The positive benefits of CBD may make you feel blissful or high on life, but CBD isn't going to get you high. It's 100 percent free of anything resembling psychoactive, psychedelic, or hallucinatory properties.

The cannabis plant, hemp's cousin, got its infamy for being a psychedelic drug. Tetrahydrocannabinol (THC), one of hundreds of chemical compounds in the plant, is responsible for creating that psychedelic experience. CBD also appears in the same plant, but it isn't nearly the same thing in form or function.

REMEMBER

Full-spectrum or broad-spectrum CBD products can have trace amounts (legally, less than 0.3 percent) of THC. That amount won't get you high, though, so as long as you're buying quality products with reputable origins and proper testing and labeling, you still don't need to worry about tripping out.

CBD Is Legal in Most States

In 2018, the United States passed the Farm Bill, making hemp a legal agricultural crop nationwide. In doing so, it technically made consuming CBD legal across the country. Although each state can pass its own laws regulating CBD consumption within its borders, only a few states have stringent CBD regulations as of this writing. Chapter 6 has details on the legalities of CBD in various states.

TIP

Check your state's government website for the most up-to-date information on local laws. A few other cannabis-centric sites, like Leafly and Weedmaps, can likely give you pretty clear direction as well, but steer clear of getting your information from single-brand sites that are looking to sell you something.

CBD Is Available from Many Sources

Because of CBD's popularity, you can pretty much find it anywhere. I'm not kidding — literally anywhere. I live in Idaho, where CBD isn't technically legal but you can find it front and center at the checkout of any number of stores. We even have stores that are specifically CBD retailers, and the signs on the sides of the building advertise that fact.

Even grocery stores these days are building out CBD sections of their aisles. You can likely find what you're looking for at most clean, environmentally focused, and responsible grocery store chains. They have to do their due diligence in vetting products for their shelves. Trusted specialty retailers and small stores are picking up CBD in droves as well. Bottom line: If a purveyor you trust is offering CBD, it may be worth a gander.

REMEMBER

If you have access to a medical or adult-use dispensary (see Chapter 6), you have more options than much of the country. Just make sure any CBD-specific retailer is selling more than a single brand. That's an excellent way to know you're exploring your options.

The internet connects you to every single brand selling CBD. Most brands have websites to sell directly to consumers, and plenty of other businesses consolidate third-party brands and sell a variety of CBD products. In fact, I own one of those stores!

You Can Take CBD Discreetly

Given all the different ways you can consume CBD (see Chapter 7), taking it as discreetly as you see fit is definitely in your control. For example, swallowing a CBD capsule is just like taking a vitamin or putting a piece of gum in your mouth. You can do it anywhere, anytime, and with incredible ease. Smoking has even become far more discreet than ever before thanks to smaller, handheld devices that can replace the more conspicuous papers, bongs, and bubblers of yesteryear. Flip to Chapter 8 for more info on consuming discreetly when necessary.

REMEMBER

Discretion is becoming a dated conversation in the CBD space thanks to CBD's increased popularity and decreased regulation. Before, consumption still felt stigmatized. Now happy newcomers and veterans alike want to share loud and proud at the top of their lungs. When I find myself an onlooker in dinner discussions where people are speculating on the benefits of CBD, I summon a bottle from my purse like the magical CBD fairy that I am. Next thing you know, everyone is adding a tincture to the top of their martinis, and happy hour just got a lot happier!

Name Brands Provide Reliability

Having legitimate companies reigning over the CBD kingdom provides not only legitimacy but also some certainty that you know what you're getting. The competency and self-regulation demanded internally by brands that intend to have some staying power in the CBD space are significant. I can speak from experience, having vetted hundreds of brands in all ways myself.

REMEMBER

Know your source. The vetting work brands are doing doesn't mean you shouldn't do your own due diligence, paying attention to what's vital for you, your body, and your health.

CBD Relieves Innumerable Conditions

Three conditions that affect Americans at an alarming rate are stress, sleeplessness, and pain. These ailments often underlie other issues as well. Stress can lead to sexual dysfunction. Insomnia can lead to a lack of focus. Pain can lead to fatigue. CBD is starting to become a key ingredient in addressing some of these symptoms and may be addressing the root causes leading to these symptoms.

Some of the more historically untreatable conditions in human health, from neurodegenerative diseases like multiple sclerosis to fibromyalgia to migraines, asthma, and arthritis, now have a glimmer of hope. CBD's numerous properties, including its anti-inflammation, antimicrobial, antifungal, neuroprotective, and pain-relieving benefits, are just what the doctor ordered. You can read more about CBD's potential applications for a variety of conditions in Part 3.

Chapter **20**

Ten Ways CBD Can Help

I n this chapter, I want to provide you with quick and simple access to all the beautiful things that CBD may help remediate in your world. The information on CBD is so broad. Sometimes distilling it down into a digestible format makes taking it all in easier.

CBD Enhances Health

In the few short years that it's been available commercially, CBD has been indicated as a treatment for a diversity of ailments and symptoms. CBD has illustrated itself as beneficial in all areas of function through what appears to be a deeply integrated connection to the body's internal processing system, the *endocannabinoid system* (see Chapter 3).

With overarching immune support thanks to its anti-inflammatory properties, CBD can address overall health and decrease so many symptoms associated with aging. Aging is a natural and inevitable process, but it's also one of the factors that most compromises feeling healthy. Pain, sleeplessness, stress, anxiety, digestive problems and so much more often become exacerbated over time. Even if these problems aren't presenting as serious conditions or even at all right now, the potential of CBD's anti-inflammatory properties to alleviate mild occurrences can help improve quality of life and overall health.

REMEMBER

CBD also has anti-depressive qualities that build on other health improvements. Whether it's actually changing your chemistry may not matter if you're just feeling better as a whole.

CBD Relieves Stress

Experiential evidence and even clinical studies are pointing to CBD as an incredible stress reliever. The body is filled almost head to toe with receptors that respond to CBD. Internally and topically, these receptors interact with CBD to lessen your stress response.

As a daily supplement, CBD can help improve your general stress response and in turn potentially minimize anxiety attacks. When consuming CBD specifically for stress and anxiety when they occur, individuals report a feeling of calm and relaxation. How quickly depends on the form of CBD used; you can read more about the forms and their onset times in Chapter 7.

CBD Controls Nausea

Nausea is caused by an imbalance between your senses and your perception and physicality. CBD as a supplemental tool has reported benefits for those experiencing nausea. A calibrated dose of CBD in the right form can also address more complex forms of nausea.

TIP

I explain CBD's applications for nausea in more detail in Chapter 11. But in general, if your nausea is a symptom of a physical experience like a boat ride, take your CBD ahead of time if possible so it has enough time to kick in. Otherwise, have a rapid-onset form on hand for nausea you can't anticipate. Check out Chapter 7 for details on which forms are best for which onset times.

CBD Relieves Pain

CBD is known as an *analgesic*, meaning that it acts to relieve pain. Furthermore, cannabis as a whole has been used since the beginning of recorded time to alleviate the pain response. Early clinical trials and all the experiential evidence around CBD in the last several years have indicated an incredible opportunity here.

Different types of pain require different types of treatment. Some may find they need topical CBD for localized acute pain, while others may need the combo of cannabis and THC to alleviate pain with chronic roots. Chapter 5 has the basics on CBD's functions for pain relief; for information on dealing with more-specific conditions with pain as a symptom, check out the chapters in Part 3.

CBD Helps You Sleep

Sleep issues are one of the most prevalent conditions that CBD helps treat and eliminate. More than a third of American adults experience sleep issues on a daily basis, ranging from restlessness to full blown insomnia.

Stress and pain are common issues that can contribute to sleeplessness, so CBD's potential for alleviating these conditions may have benefits for sleep as well. The anti-inflammatory properties of CBD have created huge opportunities for more sufferers to find a deeper night's rest.

REMEMBER

As those who are suffering from sleeplessness know, the lack of rest only contributes to amplifying whatever's keeping them from sleeping in the first place. When CBD can serve a role in helping remediate that symptom, relief is on the way. Symptoms aside, CBD seems to be helping address sleeplessness all around. Studies have indicated the CBD helps decrease cortisol levels, which contribute to sleep challenges from falling asleep to staying asleep. In high doses, CBD, through its cortisol reduction, can act as a sedative.

CBD Relieves Digestive Problems

Inflammation in the gut is one of the largest challenges to overcome in treating digestive issues. CBD can help address some contributing factors, like anxiety and pain. However, treating the side effects of these symptoms can sometimes provide the most relief in the immediate term.

REMEMBER

The anti-inflammatory properties of CBD can potentially work wonders. They can balance an inflamed gut and the gastrointestinal (GI) system and help heal the inflammatory immune response in this crucial operating system.

An added benefit is the fact that CBD lowers cortisol levels in the body and can address intestinal permeability. *Intestinal permeability* allows nutrients and other consumed matter to leak into your system, resulting in an increased and unnecessary immune response. By reducing cortisol levels through CBD consumption and addressing previous inflammatory trauma, digestion, and associated problems, you can find a sense of relief.

In situations like these, taking a form of CBD that immediately touches the GI tract is valuable. Consuming a supplemental form that dissolves in the mouth (such as a tincture or sublingual oil) is a surefire way to get CBD into the bloodstream and then the GI tract.

CBD Supports Autoimmune Treatments

An *autoimmune* condition is a case of mistaken identity where the body attacks itself. These conditions are largely difficult to treat; often, medicine treats the symptoms without being able to address immune function as a whole. Autoimmune conditions are traditionally treated with doses of anti-inflammatories on a regular schedule, so moving to CBD is a swift shift.

CBD also interacts directly with the immune system through the endocannabinoid system, which has a strong presence in immune function. Some studies have indicated that CBD can even help suppress immune dysfunction. Head to Chapter 10 for more on CBD and the immune system, as well as treating specific autoimmune conditions with CBD.

CBD Is Effective for Neurological Conditions

Thanks to the U.S. government's patent for and approval of the CBD-derived anti-seizure drug Epidiolex, I can confidently say that CBD offers effective treatments for neurological conditions. The antioxidant effects CBD has provide the claim to fame here. Oxidative stress (see Chapter 9) of tissue in the nervous system is a key contributor to neurological conditions, and as an antioxidant CBD can combat it.

REMEMBER

Seizures are only one example. Neurological conditions are far broader ranging, from Huntington's disease to dementia and more.

CBD Eases Cancer Symptoms

What's common about all types of cancer is pain and decreased immune function. With those come a whole host of other symptoms, like stress and anxiety, and potential side effects from treatment.

When cancer attacks your body, the stress imparted to all parts of your body demands an inflammatory response. The potential for CBD to reduce that inflammatory response and help remediate the body's reactions to that stress is really important.

In scenarios like these, high doses of CBD to help remediate the symptoms of the cancer itself as well as the side effects of the treatments are valuable opportunities. However, patients need to check with their doctors and treatment providers about potential drug interactions between CBD and the treatments they're already receiving.

CBD Can Help Pets, Too

You know that bumper sticker about how pets are people, too? Pets suffer from so many of the same conditions and ailments that humans do and can benefit from CBD's applications for those conditions. CBD isn't indicated in any way to be toxic or intoxicating for pets. They just require different doses based on their generally smaller size, and maybe a few different flavors like bacon tinctures and peanut butter treats. I cover CBD for pets in Chapter 15.

Chapter 21

Ten Ways to Get CBD into Your System

CBD has come a long, long way. It initially hit the scene almost exclusively in extract form. Now, several years later, it's coming full circle back to the full plant and flower form. If you can imagine a way of consuming CBD, it probably exists. The following sections highlight ten options; head to Chapter 7 for details on the variety of CBD delivery methods.

Eat a Product Containing It

I bet that if I wanted to replace almost everything in my pantry with an edible containing CBD, I very well could. Some of the earliest treats and edibles to the CBD marketplace were gummies and chocolates. These options were likely pulled directly from the THC space, which gets much of its traction in the recreational market. But the value of the CBD market is almost exclusively therapeutic, and that makes it a little bit different.

Chocolates and gummy forms are still popular, but many people looking to improve their health are going for edibles that have a more healthful spin to them. Granolas, trail mix, protein bars, nut butters, and different kinds of honey are among the new wave of options. Therapeutic applications require a degree of comfort in consumption, though, so you can still find plenty of CBD junk foods and snacks, like cookies and lollipops.

Smoke It

Being a big fan of rituals, ceremonies, and processes, I tend to love a beautiful smokable cured hemp CBD flower over almost anything else. I think I enjoy the process almost as much as I enjoy smoking it: using my fingers to break up the buds over a grinder, tearing my rolling paper in half (because I don't like to smoke more paper than I have to), laying my ground flower across the crease in the paper, and using both hands to gently roll and compact my own little personal joint. Everything about the process is a moment of personal peace and tranquility to me, which is precisely why I need CBD — to bring me much-needed stress and anxiety release.

Whether you value diverse terpene profiles, an indoor growing climate, or an outdoor one, the world is your oyster in terms of the whole-flower market. You can also choose from a great number of *pre-rolls,* where a company rolls the flower for you and you simply pull it out of a container to smoke. If you're going the pre-roll route, look for a label that says "whole flower."

TIP

Paper is a great vehicle for smoking, but don't dismiss pipes, bubblers, and bongs. Not only have they improved on their functionality over many years, but they're also incredibly attractive. With so many colorful and handblown glass options, you may be inclined to leave them on your coffee table.

Vape It

What a crazy cool market. I know, I know, vapes have gotten a bad rap. But vape cartridges come from any number of companies in regulated medical and adult-use dispensaries around the country as well as on a national open market. (You can read more about dispensaries and the open market in Chapter 6.)

REMEMBER

Make sure you trust your retailer. Vape cartridges aren't the kind of thing you want to buy at a corner store or a gas station.

So many cool vape devices are available if you need fast-acting, discreet, and maybe even vapor-free action. The standard pen cartridge with a battery is available far and wide. Stick to the metal, glass, and silicon models for safe consumption.

Dab It

Dabbing is for high doses and fast action. It's generally more appealing in the cannabis THC space but may be useful for people looking to CBD for chronic pain relief and remediation from much more serious conditions.

REMEMBER

Consuming this form not only brings on potentially intense sensations of drowsiness but can also create a significant body high. A *body high* is characterized as body-wide relaxation and mental clarity (versus a head high associated with THC cannabis) and can last as long as three hours after its immediate onset.

The appeal of dabbing, like other inhalation methods, is the quick onset and the highest *bioavailability* (the body's ability to absorb the chemical). You get the same results for less CBD (or more results for more CBD, depending on your need). The dab device is a little more complicated than those for other forms of consumption, requiring a glass piece and a butane torch. Adaptations have included dab pens, but they aren't nearly as efficient.

Smooth It on Your Skin

From pain patches to anti-aging serums, the topical CBD market has a whole spectrum of forms to choose from, including

>> Transdermal patches

>> Balms, salves, and lotions

>> Roll-ons

>> Sprays

>> Serums and oils

The two umbrella categories here are body care and skincare. Body care products are highly focused on inflammation, muscle recovery, and pain. The skincare market is largely concerned with addressing skin stress from an anti-aging perspective. The skincare space in particular is seeing some really interesting and complementary ingredient combinations. To be competitive in the beauty and skincare marketplace, brands and products have to keep evolving and building innovative formulations. Skincare is far too complex for any one product to rest on its laurels with CBD as its single highlighted ingredient.

Put It in Your Food

Adding CBD to your food seems like a no-brainer because so many CBD products are contained in a form of oil. That's most often medium-chain triglyceride (MCT) oil, a refined form of coconut oil. MCT is a popular CBD carrier oil because of its complementary benefits with CBD and its pretty much flavorless nature. Because they don't have an overwhelming flavor profile but still contain CBD, MCT-based sublingual products make the perfect additive to almost any recipe. I don't suggest cooking with CBD products, though, because they're temperature-sensitive. You don't want to kill off all the valuable plant chemicals before you've had a chance to ingest them.

TIP

Just drizzling a straightforward CBD sublingual oil across your scrambled eggs or adding it to your salad dressing is simple and easy and can provide you with the dose you need. Some cool new companies are making form factors specifically designed for just that purpose, like CBD olive oil. I had a favorite lemon-flavored (limonene and, linalool terpene-rich) MCT-based CBD oil that was amazing on top of a dessert. Think chocolate torte or ice cream. Chapter 16 has some other easy ideas for incorporating CBD into your food.

Take a Mint

Mints have the benefits of portability, ease of use, and familiarity. You can just throw them in your pocket to pull out when you feel like you need them. And they have the benefits of a sublingual (see the later section "Drop It under Your Tongue") when consumed properly. You don't chew these mints; you suck on them to allow the blood vessels under your tongue to absorb the CBD.

This form, while a little harder to produce and scarcer on the open market, has evolved enough to provide products for a variety of needs; sleep mints, stress mints, digestive mints, and just plain supplemental mints are all options.

Swallow a Pill

Capsules don't have the bioavailability of a lot of other forms, but they still have quite a bit of appeal because of their familiarity. Plenty of soft gels and gel caps are available on the market. Some are just plain CBD in a carrier oil; some are full-spectrum or broad-spectrum, and others have myriad other beneficial ingredients to help support whatever condition they're trying to treat.

TIP

I also think a pill format is pretty appealing for people struggling with sleep considerations. Popping a pill before bed and not having to worry about brushing your teeth again is quite easy. Because staying asleep throughout the night can be more of a challenge than just getting to sleep, the late release of a pill may be just right.

REMEMBER

Some conditions even require layering two different products to get the benefits of their different onset times and durations. Edibles (see the earlier section "Eat a Product Containing It") are often the choice for a later-onset layer, but a pill can serve the same purpose.

Drop It under Your Tongue

Aside from inhalables, sublinguals are the fastest, easiest, and most bioavailable in many circumstances. For all these reasons, they've become my go-to and the form factor I recommend most. Smoking just doesn't have the same level of convenience, or the comfort for people looking to remediate medical concerns. From a health perspective and an alternative medicine perspective, sublingual oils and tincture formats are tried and true.

The act of releasing a dropper full of oil or alcohol-based medicine is so simple, but it also provides a ritual of repetition that can make it just right for incorporating it into a routine. Almost every CBD brand on the market has at least one tincture, so you're bound to find the right one for you.

Drink a Beverage That Contains It

One of the oldest forms of hemp flower consumption is tea. Years ago, I encountered this incredible 90-year-old woman in a village in Mexico. When I revealed that I was in the cannabis business, she told me that her grandmother used to prepare cannabis flower tea to help her sleep at night when she was young. Much of that history has died with the elders, but any moment I get to hear a little piece of the legacy, I feel so blessed.

Teas are tried and true, but more sophisticated combinations of ingredients and bases create everything from CBD bubbly water to CBD-infused coffee. The ingredients on some of these products fall between beneficial and decadent. Sometimes certain flavors are just nice to enjoy because you've come to like the taste.

Chapter **22**

Ten Tips for Having a Great CBD Experience

Not only do you have to find the right medicine, but you also have to take it properly for maximum efficacy. Something I've learned from the cannabis space and all surrounding plant medicines is the concept of set and setting. People don't always consider the *set* (your mindset) and *setting* (the environment where you're consuming) pieces of the puzzle as thoroughly as they do what they're actually consuming. But these factors actually have just as much importance. In this chapter, I dive more deeply into what exactly set and setting mean beyond the literal definitions of the words.

REMEMBER

The set and setting concept often comes up in the context of psychedelic drug experiences. It has expanded to apply to the CBD experience even though, as I note throughout the book, CBD is not psychedelic.

Recognizing That CBD Can Help

The first step to having a successful experience with CBD is having a general recognition that it can be helpful. Knowledge and intention are powerful tools. Studies specifically around the placebo effect have shown that people taking medications with an understanding of what those medications are intended to do have up to 30 percent more success compared to those taking the same medications without any knowledge of their intended benefits.

Understanding not just the symptoms of what you're trying to treat but also their root causes is also valuable. Start with a formula like X = Y, or X + X = Y. "I have stress that may be caused by outside stressors like work and home life, but hormonal shifts may a factor as well. I intend to take a CBD sublingual daily to help alleviate my feeling of stress."

TIP

Chapter 20 provides a quick breakdown of some ways CBD can help, and I discuss a variety of CBD's potential benefits throughout the book.

Researching before Buying

The nature of the CBD marketplace is actually quite sophisticated. You have every opportunity as the consumer to explore more information on most of these products just like you can on almost anything else you consume. Because of the lack of regulation in the cannabis and CBD space, brands hold each other to a high standard of accessibility and complete transparency. The end goal is to build consumer trust and confidence.

TIP

A quick internet search will likely lead you directly to a company offering a product intended to remedy what you're trying to treat. If that's just too complicated and you're not finding what you need, email me. I've made it my business to make this plant and incredible medicine as accessible as possible. My email is BLB@shop-Poplar.com.

Make sure you can find a certificate of authenticity (COA) readily available on the product you're going to buy. The COA outlines the details of the CBD and other cannabinoids as determined by a third-party lab. If what you see on the COA doesn't back up what you see on the label, halt immediately. There's no need to dive deeper into a company that's not offering transparency when so many other companies are. You can read more about COAs in Chapter 6.

Better yet, several highly qualified marketplaces sell well-vetted products. Why not simply vet the marketplace that carries a range of products for your condition and let it do the heavy lifting for you? Searching an entire brand website can be difficult, and though I want to believe in the integrity of all of these brands, their end goal is to sell a product so they can keep up operations. That's not to say that the same isn't true of marketplaces, but at least the diligent research on the quality of the products is on their shoulders. Here are a few options:

>> `www.shop-Poplar.com`: The Eden for pain, stress, and sleep, carrying CBD and other complementary plant medicine products with experts to guide your process and complimentary discovery calls for deeper direction. It even lists a phone number you can call with an actual human on the other end of the phone.

>> `www.directcbdonline.com`: Providing, in the company's words, "natural alternatives to help you on your journey to living well and being well." It sells a wide selection of CBD-focused products with more than 100 brands.

>> `www.missgrass.com`: A female-focused THC and CBD cannabis marketplace with a selection of notable brands. It educates on all things cannabis-related, from culture to products.

Buying the Best Product

The "best" is quite relative in CBD, but it should have a pretty standard starting point. For one, the products need to have a COA (see Chapter 6). The formulations should be specific to the condition you're treating.

Start by looking at a brand's website for other ingredients that it highlights in its formulations. It should spotlight them in a way that calls attention — that is, you should be able to easily locate a term like "highlighted ingredients" or "active ingredients." Whether these ingredients are complementary or just supportive, you should be able to find a few beyond just CBD if a product is worthy. For instance, a pain-relieving topical may include arnica and turmeric. A sleep aid may include a concentration of other cannabinoids as well as melatonin or chamomile.

Look for a brand that seems serious and committed to its craft. Here are a couple of considerations:

>> **Some degree of growth can assure that the company is sticking around and can afford to back itself up in its claims and formulations.** A marketplace or large e-commerce retailer with multiple brands is likely not going to sell CBD products from brands that don't produce in huge volume as well.

>> **Quality branding, concise education, and real transparency are characteristics of good brands in the space.** Companies that present these things likely have intelligent formulations with complementary ingredients that speak to specific conditions.

REMEMBER

Price isn't always an indicator of quality. It can be, with really high quality formulations and immaculate branding. But sometimes it just means a more expensive team behind the scenes or fancier packaging.

Choosing the Form That Suits You

When you find the root condition you're addressing, check in with yourself to determine which form you think is the best for you. Are you a habitually driven person? Is picking up new habits and carrying them forward easy for you, or do you struggle to bring something into your life in a routine way without a reminder? This area may be your single most important line of self-questioning.

If the condition that you're treating is reminder enough to use a new remedy, then you have a multitude of form factors to choose from. If you find yourself starting a strong supplement regimen and then three days later forgetting about it, your best bet is probably to choose a form that you can integrate into a routine that's already part of your day. Chapter 7 has the lowdown on the various forms of CBD. Head to Chapter 8 for some examples of stacking CBD usage with existing habits.

REMEMBER

Some conditions limit your form choices a bit. For example, acute pain, migraines, and other issues that come one quickly require a quick response time. In these cases you're limited to something that's inhalable or, if you have a few more minutes, sublingual. Sleep conditions and chronic pain that can require higher concentrations and longer durations often find benefits from layering different form factors. Edibles and gel caps take longer to activate in the system, but they also last longer.

TIP

If you're supplementing with CBD for overall benefits rather than trying to relieve a specific condition, let your taste buds guide your form choice.

Finding the Proper Dose

The dosing is just as important as the form and intended function of your product. Without the proper dose and consistent use, you can't accurately judge the success. Most brands have addressed dosing for you on a fairly rudimentary level by setting standards across the industry for a baseline dose. Conversations around more complicated dosing have begun in the industry as well, but it's still not that straightforward.

Dosing is all about starting low and going slow until you find the right number of milligrams for your body. Chapter 6 has details on adjusting your dose, but I suggest you start with no more than 10 milligrams of CBD in a dose or ingestion. You can take several smaller doses a day if you choose as long as they add up to no more than 10 milligrams total and are evenly spaced throughout a single day when you are first starting out. Then, if you don't feel your intended results, you can slowly increase that dose size every three days, until you find the right dose for you.

Determining the Best Way to Buy

REMEMBER

Ultimately, the best way to buy is the one that suits your needs specifically.

If you want ongoing delivery to your doorstep, this route is simple enough. Companies often offer additional discounts for that style of loyalty, membership, or subscription. Just make sure you've dialed in the right product for you first; a subscription doesn't really serve you if it's delivering a product that doesn't do what you need. On the other hand, I prefer subscriptions because I tend to be a tad forgetful. I love a regular supply of CBD but only remember to shop when my bottles are empty. And then I have to wait until I get around to placing an online order and make do until the shipment arrives.

Some companies, like Poplar, offer concierge-style services that help you find the right product or products and create bundled regular deliveries. That's an easy way to get in tune with your needs and get your products as you need them.

If you're more of a localist and you like patronizing a certain store that carries a product you like, by all means, shop local. If it doesn't carry what you like, my guess is that it'd be interested to hear what works for you. In my experience, customer feedback drives a good business model, and your store may just pick up your favorite brand.

Being in a Good Physical Space

I believe knowing what physical spaces make you feel comfortable and creating that setting for yourself is really important. You might say you're "setting" yourself for success. By finding a space where you're going to enjoy the process and really sink into the good you're intending to provide yourself, you improve your chances for success. In my opinion, an optimal environment gives your body the best chance of vibing with your supplement of choice.

Because everybody is different and the form factors vary so widely, you're going to find a great degree of variability in setting. Medicinal use of plant medicine has traditionally taken place in very curated environments with ceremonies and rituals at the heart of the process. Every piece of a ceremony is very intimately selected to improve the outcome. CBD use is more supplemental and can be every day, so I don't think you need to go so far as to create a ceremony every time you use it unless you want to. You may want to consider how you can ritualize the process to make consumption more enjoyable.

If you already have a comforting ritual, like drinking your morning beverage, you can incorporate CBD use into that setting. I like to give myself a little verbal reminder of what I'm doing and why I'm doing it. You can say something like, "Every time I take this tincture, I feel calmer and more relaxed." You can say it out loud like an affirmation, whisper it mentally — whatever works for you. Establishing that intention in a consistent setting day over day provides better results and more follow-through than you may imagine.

Getting Your Head Right

What could be a better way to get your head right than talking about intention and ritual? Your presence right here, right now, reading about CBD already illustrates a degree of curiosity, mindfulness, and self-awareness. Fortunately, that makes my job a little bit easier. CBD can really help the noise and busyness around you fade into the background, creating even more presence and self-awareness.

Adding a Complementary Product

You can boost the sensations of CBD in many ways. Here are a few options:

TIP

>> If you're looking for overall immune support and supplementation, stack some *functional mushrooms* (specific types of mushrooms with medicinal benefits) into your routine. These days they come in all sorts of forms, from ground coffee to canned beverages with cacao, turmeric, and matcha.

Four Sigmatic makes a great ground coffee blend with functional mushrooms. For a variety of yummy CBD-infused beverages in this category, check out Earth and Star.

>> If you're taking CBD for a mood boost, layer it with anything cacao, which has *anandamide,* the joy molecule. For the most part, I'm talking about beautiful, deep, dark, raw cacao here, not the stuff you get out of vending machines. You can also buy sipping cacao and make a beverage that tastes much like hot chocolate but has far more beneficial properties for your body.

>> Skincare regimens that layer complementary products tend to offer enhanced results. Apple cider vinegar (ACV) serums, facial moisturizers, or *hydrosols* (a water byproduct of essential oil production) can be great complements to any number of CBD skincare products.

Trying Something New When You Feel Comfortable

When you've gotten the hang of one product, you may be ready to try another. Maybe you're highly novelty-seeking and think diversity is the spice of life. That's great! Maybe you want to experiment with different forms for another reason. My biggest suggestion to you here is to find your initial "correct" dose (see the earlier section "Finding the Proper Dose" and Chapter 6) and apply that same methodology to whatever you pick up next.

REMEMBER

Not all CBD products are created equally. Different complementary ingredients may change the way your body interacts with the medicine. Additionally, the onset time and bioavailability may change based on your consumption method. So although 10 milligrams seems like 10 milligrams universally, it's not quite the same. For example, a chocolate bar may have an earlier onset and a stronger result than swallowing a capsule.

If you want to try a form with a quicker onset than what you've had previously, you'll likely switch to smokables. The sensation is almost always going to be more intense and immediate. Be prepared. It's not going to last as long, so you may want to consider a smaller dose when you're first starting and see how you feel. Too high a dose for too long a duration can be a little bit of a shock to the system.

Appendix **A**

Helpful CBD Resources

Sometimes, opening the door into a new knowledge base inspires a hunger for more knowledge. Additionally, the field of CBD research is so new that new information on best practices and uses for CBD flows constantly, so I want to make sure you have all the evolving resources at your fingertips. In this appendix, I share some of my favorite resources, from websites to organizations that are getting ahead of curve.

REMEMBER

This appendix isn't exhaustive. I've left out a lot of sources that tend to be too business-focused for what I cover in this book. Here, I focus on the safe and updated what, why, and how of CBD!

Resources for Using CBD

When you're exploring information about CBD in terms of health and wellness, CBD is CBD is CBD. It serves the same purpose no matter what country you live in, and the scientific information on the plant chemical is the same. The following sections include some of the more accessible and informative sources of information that cover the use of CBD regardless of where you live.

TIP

For details about legality outside the United States, I suggest you explore resources that are in your country. The later section "Updated CBD Guidelines" has some options that may be able to help with that.

Know Your CBD (International)

www.knowyourcbd.info

I love this site, but I may be a bit partial. I've partnered with it to be one of the go-to experts for providing information. In an attempt to unify cohesive information in the space, brands and cannabis advocates got together to share information in bite-size nuggets. How, what, when, why, and so forth are in there, all from trusted industry experts and partners.

CBD Resource (U.K.-based)

www.cbdresource.co.uk

This European educational blog is a useful source for articles on news and education in the CBD space. It has sections on how-to guides, fun facts, and even other cannabinoids.

Informative CBD Websites

With the internet at your fingertips, you have more resources available than anyone could imagine. I highly recommend sticking to this whole reference guide as your resource guide, at least for the foreseeable future. Because of the lack of research and the fact that the industry is still evolving, brands still largely control and distribute information about CBD. That wouldn't necessarily be so much of a challenge if brands didn't have an agenda, but unfortunately not all are trustworthy. Here's a couple sites worth a look-see.

Project CBD

www.projectcbd.org

This site has been a resource in the industry since 2009. It's a California-based nonprofit created by journalists to share the story of medical cannabis. It relates what's happening in the industry as well as relevant science. The "Resources" section has what it calls "educational brochures" that you may find helpful. The content may not be continually updated, but it can be a good place to start.

Be Poplar

www.be-poplar.com

This site is an educational blog on wellness. While it covers a host of use scenarios for CBD and other wellness products, it also touches on products that speak to addressing those use cases. If you need more information to get your CBD journey started, please reach out to us at Poplar for a free consultation with me: https://shop-poplar.com/pages/book-a-free-consultation.

You can also email us with specific questions: help@shop-poplar.com.

TIP

This site also has a shop (www.shop-poplar.com). Here's a discount coupon you can use there for 20 percent off your first purchase with Poplar. Please use the code *Dummies*.

Industry-Focused Hemp Information

hempindustrydaily.com

This online publication is a part of MJBiz Daily, one of the largest and more reputable cannabis resources in the industry. It also has a section-by-section opportunity to explore not only every U.S. state but also internationally as well. Check out the "By Region" section for details.

Informative Cannabis Resources

CBD is just one piece to the cannabis plant, and, cohesive resources supporting it aren't quite as available as cannabis resources are. However, cannabis resources can provide good, reliable information on CBD.

REMEMBER

Because these sites are largely focused on cannabis as a whole, they cover THC heavily as well. Many may also be proponents of the opinion that CBD is only effective with the presence of THC. This entire book indicates otherwise, so if you aren't interested in THC or other cannabinoids, you still have a great option in CBD.

Leafly (U.S.-based)

https://www.leafly.com/

This site was designed to help you access legal cannabis in your state across the United States. It provides details on brands, where they're available, and the ability to order cannabis when it's legal. So if you're looking for more info or for specific cannabis-derived or hemp-derived CBD, you can find brand and strain-specific information, including where and how to get it.

Weed Maps (U.S.-based)

http://weedmaps.com/

This site was created to offer a map on cannabis retail outlets in the United States, but it has evolved to share pertinent information on different strains of cannabis, including hemp strains. This source is one of the best places to go to understand flower and all the various properties of specific flower strains.

Miss Grass

missgrass.com/blogs/basics

Miss Grass is the coolest lady-focused cannabis content provider (and retailer for the United States). Created as a timely representation of what the world of legal cannabis entails, it also covers a fair number of CBD topics with relevancy and a great tone. Even if you are not interested in trying THC cannabis, you can learn a lot about the legal market and the whens, whys, and hows.

Hello MD

hellomd.com/tag/cbd

Hello MD, a company focused on providing medical marijuana prescriptions in the United States, has done a beautiful job providing a wealth of knowledge on CBD-related concerns. So if you are U.S.-based and need a script to access cannabis-derived CBD from a medical dispensary, start here for your medical access card, and then explore the site's information database including recommendations and recipes.

Cannabis Health (U.K.-based)

www.cannabishealthnews.co.uk

This U.K.-based publication on European cannabis shares details on cannabis medicine and the well-being space from a variety of angles. Lots of what it covers is CBD-centric. Because the legality of CBD is much broader than cannabis as a whole across Europe, the site also seems to do a great job covering European legal considerations. Like other, more traditional print publications also living online, it does have lots of ads. Just recognize that these are companies paying to promote among validated press and industry news rather than endorsements from the publication itself.

Trade Organizations

Here are my favorite national and international cannabis associations and organizations. For the most part, they aren't hemp-specific. Some are, and some are more general to botanicals and herbs. Most are specific to policy, access, and social justice — the important pieces!

Hemp Industries Association (HIA)

thehia.org/

This organization has been around longer than most of the cannabis organizations of note because hemp was in demand for industrial purposes long before cannabis for consumption came back into fashion. Education and integrity are the focus of HIA.

Drug Policy Alliance

drugpolicy.org/

One of the most, if not the most, respected organizations working toward advancing perception and policy in the cannabis space. The focus of its messaging is harm reduction in use and prohibition while supporting individuals.

Marijuana Policy Project

www.mpp.org/

Founded in 1995, this organization is focused on reforming U.S. marijuana laws through lobbying, press initiatives, and industry coalitions, among other things. Its focus has been on removing criminal penalties for use and medical availability for patients. It does great work.

Law Enforcement Action Partnership (LEAP)

lawenforcementactionpartnership.org/

Founded in early 2002, this nonprofit is made up of current and former members of the law enforcement and criminal justice communities. They call themselves "the new voice of criminal justice reform," recognizing the negative impacts the War on Drugs had on communities of color. They are taking education and the advancement of justice into their own hands.

American Herbal Pharmacopoeia (AHP)

herbal-ahp.org/

This organization is dedicated to promoting the responsible use of herbal products and herbal medicines.

Americans For Safe Access

www.safeaccessnow.org/

Americans For Safe Access is one of the most respected cannabis organizations in the industry. Its mission: "advancing medical and cannabis therapeutics and research." Advocacy across medical use through policy and lawmaking is a priority. This organization is very important for cannabis and CBD, but it is a little more industry-centric.

American Trade Association for Cannabis & Hemp (ATACH)

atach.org/

Designed to promote the expansion, protection, and preservation of the cannabis industry as a whole, ATACH doesn't limit its work to just cannabis. It also covers hemp-based products across industrial, recreational, and medical spaces.

Cannabis Trade Federation (CTF)

www.cannabistradefederation.com/

Many challenges face the cannabis industry from a foundational standpoint. CTF focuses on participating in making these challenges more manageable. Its priorities include diversity and inclusion, eliminating the challenges of the state and federal inconsistencies with illegality, and helping with making banking a possibility for these companies.

Cannabis Canada Association

http://cmcia.ca/

This organization (originally known as the Canadian Medical Cannabis Industry Association) is a member-driven association for licensed producers of medical cannabis in Canada, but it actually has some good, quality information on the use of CBD.

Conferences

I'd love to suggest a whole host of events that you can explore, but at this juncture they're so niche that it's going to be hard to offer cohesive direction. The best thing to do is to search your area for events on hemp and on CBD and then validate them by checking to see their organizational affiliations or even their expert alliances. Most of the big events are tied to industry needs like production, growing, processing, branding, and investing.

MJ Biz Con (U.S.-based)

mjbizconference.com

It's the largest cannabis conference in the world! From investors to executives, this conference has been connecting over 30,000 cannabis enthusiasts since 2011. It's a cannabis-centric event that also has an online virtual event, and now sections of the event are specifically dedicated to hemp and CBD. However, if you're just consuming CBD, this conference may be a little too industry-focused for you.

NoCo Hemp Expo (U.S.-based)

www.nocohempexpo.com

Covering business, farming, and investment in the hemp space, this expo is held annually. Though it pales in comparison to the size of MJ Biz Con (see the preceding section), it's specifically focused on hemp, including considerations around hemp as an industrial commodity and food source, and has the potential to grow significantly as the industry grows.

Informative CBD Science Articles

If you're inclined to dig a little deeper, here are the two places you need to go to find available research on CBD.

REMEMBER

To be validated by the scientific community in the Western medical world, information has to be *peer-reviewed,* a process where medical professionals evaluate information for validity, which can take as long as a year. So from research (sometimes years) to writing (more time) to publishing (even more time), this information takes a while to land somewhere you can access it, by which point it may not be the most up-to-date. I believe this format works for the Western medical world but also that Eastern cultures have been using cannabis in particular as medicine with success for generations. So I like to cross over all this information to stay timely and effective.

Journal of Cannabis Research

jcannabisresearch.biomedcentral.com/

An official publication of the Institute of Cannabis Research, this peer-reviewed medical journal publishes all aspects of cannabis research, including but not limited to cannabis pharmacology, clinical and preclinical information, public health considerations, cannabis-related disorders, the endocannabinoid system, and more. This journal is an important resource for me and my peers for understanding cannabis as a whole and as it relates to use cases with the human body. CBD is a big part of that. So though it may be a bit broader than you may need, this source is the place to go if you really want to embrace your inner nerd!

PubMed

https://pubmed.ncbi.nlm.nih.gov/

More generally, this site is my go-to resource for all medical applications and conditions. It's a compilation of millions of references to biomedical literature. Maintained by the Center for Biotechnology Information (NCBI) and the U.S. National Library of Medicine (NLM), it's one of the most, if not the most, comprehensive sources online for biomedicine and health. I cross reference my searches here, and though it may be a little too science-y for some, each article has an intro that provides an *abstract* (a synopsis and summary of the information). You can easily search your condition in the search browser of this site for a little deeper dive into your considerations and needs. I love to geek out online with all its information.

Updated CBD Guidelines

Legality around CBD isn't a certain thing on any given day. Laws are changing regularly and you're responsible as a consumer for knowing whether what you're doing is legal. Here's a list of great resources to know what you can and can't do, state-by-state in the United States and country-by-country around the world.

Daily CBD

dailycbd.com/en/

Offering a worldwide map, Daily CBD created a searchable platform to explore the legality of CBD as well as the products available in your region. For buyers outside the United States, this site may be the best starting point to know what you can access. From my experience, I can say that its information about legality on a country-by-country basis and its how-to's are relevant, though I can't testify to the quality of the product recommendations.

U.S. Food and Drug Administration (U.S.-based)

www.fda.gov/news-events/public-health-focus/fda-regulation-cannabis-and-cannabis-derived-products-including-cannabidiol-cbd

The FDA provides the United States's version of guidelines for regulation regarding the safety and effectiveness of biological products and devices (primarily food and cosmetics) for humans and animals.

REMEMBER

The FDA isn't the regulating body, so in an unregulated space like CBD, it can share perceptions and interpretations of regulations until formal laws are passed.

Health Canada

www.canada.ca/en/health-canada/services/drugs-medication/cannabis/about/cannabidiol.html

Health Canada is a country-regulated website that indicates the legal standing in Canada of cannabis and hemp and thus CBD. This URL gives you access to all the legal information you need to navigate what you can and can't do within the country to stay safe and aboveboard.

The European Commission

https://ec.europa.eu/search/?queryText=cannabinoid&query_source=europa_default&filterSource=europa_default&swlang=en&more_options_language=en&more_options_f_formats=*&more_options_date=*

The European regulator for the markets is the European Commission. This URL directs you specifically to a search on cannabinoids, because I must admit, it's a little hard to navigate unless you know exactly what you're looking for. Try a few different keywords in the search browser.

Index

Numbers

2018 Farm Bill, 60, 261

A

acne, 168
adaptogenic botanicals, 56
addictions, 159–161
adult-use dispensary, 63
adverse reactions, 55–56
aging, 166–167
Agriculture Improvement Act of 2018, 60, 261
AHP (American Herbal Pharmacopoeia), 290
alcohol
  addiction to, 160–161
  as base for sublinguals, 87
  recipes with, 219–226
Alger, Bradley, 34
Alzheimer's disease, 108–109
American Herbal Pharmacopoeia (AHP), 290
American Sleep Association, 49
American Trade Association for Cannabis & Hemp (ATACH), 290–291
Americans For Safe Access, 290
analgesic, 266
anandamide, 158, 176
anorexia, 132–135
anxiety
  eating disorders and, 135–136
  Huntington's disease and, 107–108
  menopause and, 179
  modulating, 156–157
  overview, 48–49
  in pets, 185–188
  stress vs., 152–155
  THC increasing, 154
  treatments for, 153–154

Aplos Margarita Mocktail, 226
apoptosis, 189
appetite
  boosting, 133–134, 189–190
  CBD and, 134
  regulating blood sugar by suppressing, 149
  THC stimulating, 132
arthritis, 51
asthma, 145–147
ATACH (American Trade Association for Cannabis & Hemp), 290–291
atopic eczema, 169
autoimmune diseases
  cannabis and, 116–117
  caused by neurological conditions, 104
  CBD and, 115–119, 268
  celiac disease, 127–129
  defined, 115
  inflammation and, 116
  lupus, 119–123
  Lyme disease, 124–126
  multiple sclerosis, 111–112
  stress and, 116–117
  terpenes and, 117–118
Awaken Arousal Oil, 182

B

balms, 83–84, 174
bath bombs, 113, 142–143, 174, 249
beta-caryophyllene, 117, 132
beverages. See also drinking CBD; recipes
  Aplos Margarita Mocktail, 226
  Bulletproof Chai with CBD, 218
  Cacao Mezcal Heart Opener, 220
  CBD Chamomile Lemonade, 213
  CBD Old-Fashioned, 222

doctors, 54–55, 260

dopamine, 33

dosing

  adjusting

    to one's needs, 69, 92–93, 96–98

    to pets, 193

  for Alzheimer's disease, 109

  for anxiety, 154

  for bath bombs, 143

  for bipolar disorder, 162–163

  for bulimia, 136–137

  for chronic fatigue syndrome, 111

  for cramps, 172

  determining, 280–281

  etiquette and, 96

  for Huntington's disease, 108

  importance of bioavailability, 94–95

  for libido, 180

  for lupus, 122

  for Lyme disease, 126

  at mealtimes, 94

  microdosing, 68, 97–98

  for migraines, 147

  for multiple sclerosis, 112–113

  overview, 92–95

  pets and, 191–193

  for PTSD, 158, 188

  scheduling, 93–94

  for sleep aid, 93–94, 97, 137

  workouts and, 94

Dravet syndrome, 190–191

drinking CBD. *See also* beverages; recipes

  cooking and, 88–89

  as delivery system, 276

  overview, 78–79

  scheduling dosing, 94

Drug Policy Alliance, 289

dryness in mouth and eyes, 121

dysmenorrhea, 171–172

E

eating CBD. *See also* cooking with CBD; recipes

  affecting bioavailability, 79

  as delivery system, 271–272

  overview, 12–13, 78–79

  scheduling dosing, 94

eating disorders. *See* disorders

echinacea, 26

ECS. *See* endocannabinoid system

eczema, 169

elasticity, skin, 166–167

electric daisy, 26

emotional disorders. *See* disorders

emotions, modulating, 156–157

Empower, 123

endocannabinoid system

  in brain, 105

  female health and, 171

  insulin and, 149

  overview, 31–34

  receptors in, 51

  topical products and, 123

entourage effect, 20

enzymes, 23, 34, 53

epilepsy, 104, 190–191

erectile dysfunction, 181

European Commission, 294

extracting CBD

  defined, 37

  forms of, 73–76

  labels and, 64–65

  methods for, 38–41

F

FDA (Food and Drug Administration), 60, 104, 293–294

Federal Food, Drug, and Cosmetic Act (FD&C), 60

federal laws, 60

fibromyalgia, 144–145
Figi, Charlotte, 191
flavonoids, 21–23, 40
Fleurmarche, 70
flowers, 20, 26, 80–81, 89
Food and Drug Administration (FDA), 60, 104, 293–294
full-spectrum CBD, 11, 39, 74, 261
functional mushrooms, 282

G

GABA-A receptor, 33
Gado Gado Salad, 230
gastrointestinal problems, 121
gels, 85
generalized anxiety disorder (GAD), 153
glioblastoma, 188
Glowing CBD Face Mask, 246
gluten in CBD products, 128
Groovy Chocolate-Covered Strawberries, 239
growing cannabis, 67–68
gummies, 201–202
Gupta, Sanjay, 191

H

hash and kief, 76
headaches, 147–148
Health Canada, 294
Helichrysum, 26
Hello MD, 288
Hemp Industries Association (HIA), 289
hemp plant
  as bioremediator, 19, 66
  cannabinoids in, 21
  cannabis vs., 65
  growing, 67–68
  nervines and, 174
  overview, 17–20
  varieties of, 23–25
hemp seed oil, 171
heroin, 160
HIA (Hemp Industries Association), 289

hippocampus, 49
Homemade Food for Your Fur Baby Plus CBD, 255
homeostasis, 29
hormones, 177
Humblebloom, 70
humulene, 117–118, 132
Huntington's disease, 106–108
hydrogels, 85
hydrosols, 85
hyperthyroidism, 121
hypothyroidism, 121

I

immune suppressant, 116
immunomodulators, 116
inflammation
  anti-inflammatory properties of CBD, 105–106
  autoimmune diseases and, 116
  of brain, 109
  CFS and, 110–111
  lupus and, 120
  neurological conditions and, 104–106
infusing CBD, 41–43, 174
ingesting CBD, 11–13, 260, 262
inhalation, 272–273
insomnia. *See* sleep
Institute of Cannabis Research, 292
insulin resistance, 148–149
intestinal permeability, 268
isolate CBD, 11, 40, 41, 75, 209

J

joints, 142–143
Journal of Cannabis Research, 292

K

kava, 27
kidney problems, 121
kief and hash, 76
Know Your CBD website, 286

L

labels, 64–67
Law Enforcement Action Partnership (LEAP), 290
Leafly, 288
leaves, 20
legality
  criminalization of, 15
  laws
    federal, 60
    state, 61–62, 261
  overview, 15–16
  pregnancy and, 175
Lemon Chia Coconut Bliss Balls, 241
Levo, 203
libido, 180
limonene, 117, 132
linalool, 117
liver problems, 121
lotions, 83–84
Lucy's No Bake Anti-Inflammatory Pumpkin Dog Treats, 254
lungs, 145–146
lupus, 119–123
Lyme disease, 124–126

M

mania, 162
manic depression, 161–163
Marijuana Policy Project, 290
MCT (medium-chain triglyceride) oil, 54, 206
medical dispensary, 63
medications
  CBD interacting with, 53, 122
  placebo effect, 277–278
  side effects of, 155–157
medicinal use of CBD, 10–11, 66–67, 263
medium-chain triglyceride (MCT) oil, 54, 206
melatonin, 45
menopause, 178–179
mental effects of CBD, 34–35
microcirculation, 84

microdosing, 68, 97–98
migraines, 147–148
mints, 274–275
Miss Grass, 70, 288
MJBiz, 287, 291
modulating emotions, 156–157
morning sickness, 138
motion sickness, 139–140
mu opioid receptors, 33
multiple sclerosis (MS), 111–114
muscles. *See also* pain
  bath bombs and, 142–143
  CBD and, 141–143
  fibromyalgia, 144–145
  menstrual cramps, 171–174
  soreness of, 142
  spasms, 126
  using hemp-derived dermal solutions, 142
myrcene, 118, 132

N

nanopartializing CBD, 40
National Library of Medicine (NLM), 293
national marketplace, 63
natural CBD, 27–28
nausea, 137–140, 266
NCBI (Center for Biotechnology Information), 293
nerve issues, 121
nervines, 56, 153, 174
neurological conditions
  Alzheimer's disease, 108–109
  autoimmune diseases caused by, 104
  CBD and, 105–106, 268
  chronic fatigue syndrome, 110–111
  Dravet syndrome, 190–191
  epilepsy, 104, 190–191
  Huntington's disease, 106–108
  inflammation and, 104–106, 109
  multiple sclerosis, 111–114
neuroprotectant, 34–35, 104
Nirvana Truffles, 243

About the Author

Blair Lauren Brown is a plant medicine veteran. With over 15 years of training across Ayurveda, Ashtanga Yogic Philosophy, and Western plant sciences, she applies a holistic philosophy to everything she touches. She is the co-founder of Poplar, a modern drugstore that provides services and products for all-natural pain relief, stress relief, sleep support, and more. Blair sources and vets every product that lands at Poplar, building an intricate knowledge of the natural drug space in the U.S. market. Poplar, in its diverse plant medicine offering, also serves legal cannabis, helping CBD veterans and newbies alike by providing clean, transparent, and effective remedies and simple pleasures.

Blair is a respected NPD (natural products developer) drawing from Eastern and Western best practices to create innovative wellness formulations. In 2016, she founded Verté Essentials, the first wellness company utilizing CBD as an active ingredient. Designed for beauty from the inside out and addressing stress on the skin caused by internal stressors, Verté Essentials as a wellness and beauty brand has been featured in *Forbes* and *Cosmopolitan,* among others.

In the last 17 years, she has refined her focus as a cannabis expert and dedicated herself to learning about and educating on the intricacies of weed. Blair's cannabis roots extend beyond her businesses, recalling her role on the ground in early 2004 assisting in medical grow operations supporting California's Prop 215. Following a path of deep appreciation for the journey of cannabis culture through prohibition to the present day, her advocacy in the space illustrates a dedication to a more progressive future. She uses her platform to destigmatize cannabis and point out the legal inequalities in the justice system surrounding cannabis possession and use. You can find out more about her philosophy in her talk for TEDxSunValley.

As an acclaimed speaker, advocating for plant medicine in the form of education, she also shares her extensive knowledge of plant medicine with a broad audience across retreats, events, Clubhouse, and more.

Dedication

This book is dedicated to my partner in crime, soul sister, and co-founder Beryl Solomon. Her contributions to the book and her compassion, understanding, and allowances during the time of writing this book are beyond my unreasonable expectations.

This book is also dedicated to the six generations of medical practitioners in my family who cultivated an interest in medicine and patient care across my entire family. To my grandfather, who opened the door to medical cannabis as a prescribing pediatrician in California. To my mother, who was his patient. To my brother, also my first teacher, guardian, and best friend, who brought me up in the cannabis space from day one and still guides me to this day. To my father, who patiently mediated my endeavors as well as my brother's as we continued to dive deeper into optimizing cannabis medicine and patient care.

This book is dedicated to my beautiful son, Rhodes, and his kind, adventure-loving father. Rhodie inherits a legacy of plant medicine from me and the discovery of the natural world around him from his father. A child of the land, with curiosity as big as the ocean and as deep as the sky. He is afforded the opportunity to be in all of that. I believe that to fully understand and work with all the beauty of plant medicine, one must have a relationship with nature. With that comes the ability to understand why it is worth conserving. His father's compassionate and supportive nature encourages that for both Rhodes and me. For that, I am truly grateful. I full-heartedly believe the best I can do for Rhodes is allow him the space to understand and appreciate the natural world by being a part of it and having reverence for that which came before him. With these tools, I believe he can be an earth-loving man and a global citizen with a deep respect for community building.

To that, none of this exploration of CBD, cannabis, or plant medicine would have been possible without all that has been afforded by those before me. The consideration and conservation of the earth and community are tremendous and require a strong foundation to build from. There are not words enough to express my gratitude for those who have been a part of building that foundation. I have been able to use, explore, and write about cannabis with encouragement and support in all directions. Those before me had limited access. People before me were criminalized, imprisoned, or worse, murdered. To those who suffered because of what I believe we all deserve unabashed access to for purposes of health and well-being, I am truly grateful.

Thank you.

Author's Acknowledgments

I would like to acknowledge each and every person who helped me articulate my knowledge and get it on paper. It took a village to get this book completed and polished into the gem that it is now! Where would I be without my wonderful editors and the team at Wiley, for bringing me into the family and helping me in this incredible process? A special thank you to Megan Knoll, Chrissy Guthrie, and Tracy Boggier! And Tracy, bet you didn't think we would get so intimate out of the gates as we started exploring the potential of this book. I am so thankful to you for opening the door and letting me in. I was also able to bring in two people very dear to me to help bring this gem to light. One of them was Amiah Taylor, a new friend and editor. Anything about my work that is crystal clear and concise, that is Amiah's brilliance and talent in helping me make my writing accessible. She is a truly gifted writer and served as a wonderful editing partner. And April Pride, a dear friend and ally in the cannabis space, made sure you were getting the real, honest-to-goodness truth about CBD. I'd like to acknowledge all their hard work and commitment to the cause because it gave me a sense of much-needed solidarity.

Thank you.

Publisher's Acknowledgments

Senior Acquisitions Editor: Tracy Boggier

Managing Editor: Kristie Pyles

Editorial Project Manager and Development Editor: Christina N. Guthrie

Copy Editor: Megan Knoll

Technical Editor: April Pride

Production Editor: Mohammed Zafar Ali

Cover Image: © Yancy Caldwell

Take dummies with you everywhere you go!

Whether you are excited about e-books, want more from the web, must have your mobile apps, or are swept up in social media, dummies makes everything easier.

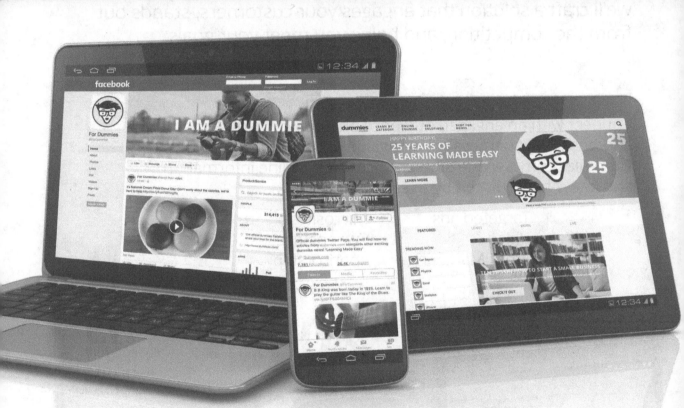

Find us online!

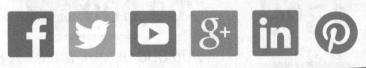

dummies.com

dummies
A Wiley Brand

Leverage the power

Dummies is the global leader in the reference category and one of the most trusted and highly regarded brands in the world. No longer just focused on books, customers now have access to the dummies content they need in the format they want. Together we'll craft a solution that engages your customers, stands out from the competition, and helps you meet your goals.

Advertising & Sponsorships

Connect with an engaged audience on a powerful multimedia site, and position your message alongside expert how-to content. Dummies.com is a one-stop shop for free, online information and know-how curated by a team of experts.

- Targeted ads
- Video
- Email Marketing
- Microsites
- Sweepstakes sponsorship

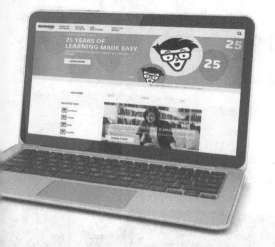

20 MILLION PAGE VIEWS EVERY SINGLE MONTH

15 MILLION UNIQUE VISITORS PER MONTH

43% OF ALL VISITORS ACCESS THE SITE VIA THEIR MOBILE DEVICES

700,000 NEWSLETTER SUBSCRIPTIONS TO THE INBOXES OF

300,000 UNIQUE INDIVIDUALS EVERY WEEK

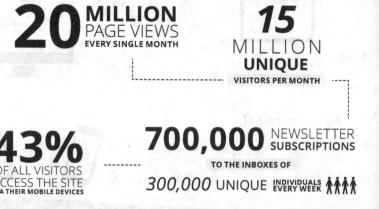

# of dummies

Custom Publishing

Reach a global audience in any language by creating a solution that will differentiate you from competitors, amplify your message, and encourage customers to make a buying decision.

- Apps
- Books
- eBooks
- Video
- Audio
- Webinars

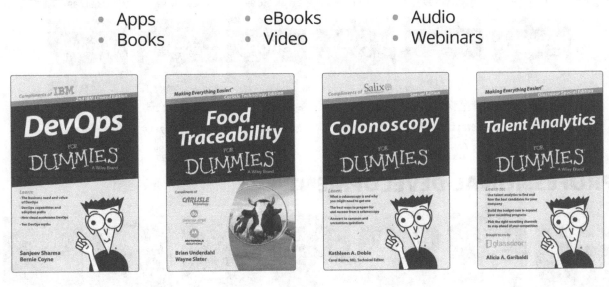

Brand Licensing & Content

Leverage the strength of the world's most popular reference brand to reach new audiences and channels of distribution.

For more information, visit dummies.com/biz

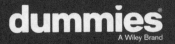

PERSONAL ENRICHMENT

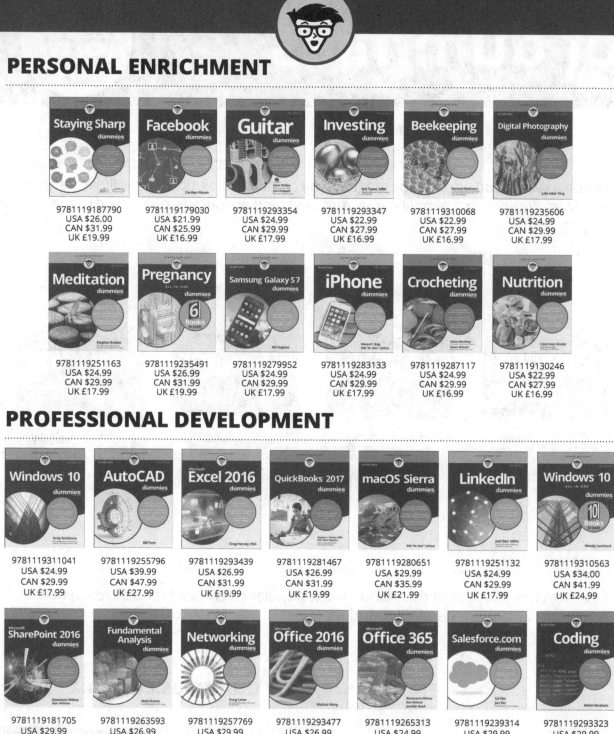

Staying Sharp dummies
9781119187790
USA $26.00
CAN $31.99
UK £19.99

Facebook dummies
Carolyn Abram
9781119179030
USA $21.99
CAN $25.99
UK £16.99

Guitar dummies
Mark Phillips, Jon Chappell
9781119293354
USA $24.99
CAN $29.99
UK £17.99

Investing dummies
Eric Tyson, MBA
9781119293347
USA $22.99
CAN $27.99
UK £16.99

Beekeeping dummies
Howland Blackiston
9781119310068
USA $22.99
CAN $27.99
UK £16.99

Digital Photography dummies
Julie Adair King
9781119235606
USA $24.99
CAN $29.99
UK £17.99

Meditation dummies
Stephan Bodian
9781119251163
USA $24.99
CAN $29.99
UK £17.99

Pregnancy ALL-IN-ONE dummies
6 Books in one
9781119235491
USA $26.99
CAN $31.99
UK £19.99

Samsung Galaxy S7 dummies
Bill Hughes
9781119279952
USA $24.99
CAN $29.99
UK £17.99

iPhone dummies
Edward C. Baig, Bob "Dr. Mac" LeVitus
9781119283133
USA $24.99
CAN $29.99
UK £17.99

Crocheting dummies
Karen Manthey, Susan Brittain
9781119287117
USA $24.99
CAN $29.99
UK £16.99

Nutrition dummies
Carol Ann Rinzler
9781119130246
USA $22.99
CAN $27.99
UK £16.99

PROFESSIONAL DEVELOPMENT

Windows 10 dummies
Andy Rathbone
9781119311041
USA $24.99
CAN $29.99
UK £17.99

AutoCAD dummies
Bill Fane
9781119255796
USA $39.99
CAN $47.99
UK £27.99

Excel 2016 dummies
Greg Harvey, PhD
9781119293439
USA $26.99
CAN $31.99
UK £19.99

QuickBooks 2017 dummies
Stephen L. Nelson, MBA, CPA, MS in Taxation
9781119281467
USA $26.99
CAN $31.99
UK £19.99

macOS Sierra dummies
Bob "Dr. Mac" LeVitus
9781119280651
USA $29.99
CAN $35.99
UK £21.99

LinkedIn dummies
Joel Elad, MBA
9781119251132
USA $24.99
CAN $29.99
UK £17.99

Windows 10 ALL-IN-ONE dummies
10 Books in one
Woody Leonhard
9781119310563
USA $34.00
CAN $41.99
UK £24.99

SharePoint 2016 dummies
Rosemarie Withee, Ken Withee
9781119181705
USA $29.99
CAN $35.99
UK £21.99

Fundamental Analysis dummies
Matt Krantz
9781119263593
USA $26.99
CAN $31.99
UK £19.99

Networking dummies
Doug Lowe
9781119257769
USA $29.99
CAN $35.99
UK £21.99

Office 2016 dummies
Wallace Wang
9781119293477
USA $26.99
CAN $31.99
UK £19.99

Office 365 dummies
Rosemarie Withee, Ken Withee, Jennifer Reed
9781119265313
USA $24.99
CAN $29.99
UK £17.99

Salesforce.com dummies
Liz Kao, Jon Paz
9781119239314
USA $29.99
CAN $35.99
UK £21.99

Coding dummies
Nikhil Abraham
9781119293323
USA $29.99
CAN $35.99
UK £21.99

dummies.com

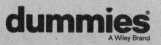

dummies
A Wiley Brand

Learning Made Easy

ACADEMIC

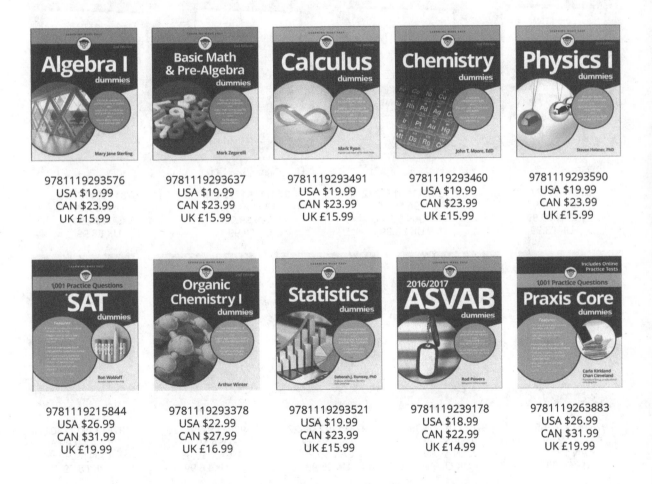

Algebra I
9781119293576
USA $19.99
CAN $23.99
UK £15.99

Basic Math & Pre-Algebra
9781119293637
USA $19.99
CAN $23.99
UK £15.99

Calculus
9781119293491
USA $19.99
CAN $23.99
UK £15.99

Chemistry
9781119293460
USA $19.99
CAN $23.99
UK £15.99

Physics I
9781119293590
USA $19.99
CAN $23.99
UK £15.99

SAT
9781119215844
USA $26.99
CAN $31.99
UK £19.99

Organic Chemistry I
9781119293378
USA $22.99
CAN $27.99
UK £16.99

Statistics
9781119293521
USA $19.99
CAN $23.99
UK £15.99

ASVAB
9781119239178
USA $18.99
CAN $22.99
UK £14.99

Praxis Core
9781119263883
USA $26.99
CAN $31.99
UK £19.99

Available Everywhere Books Are Sold

dummies.com

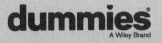

Small books for big imaginations

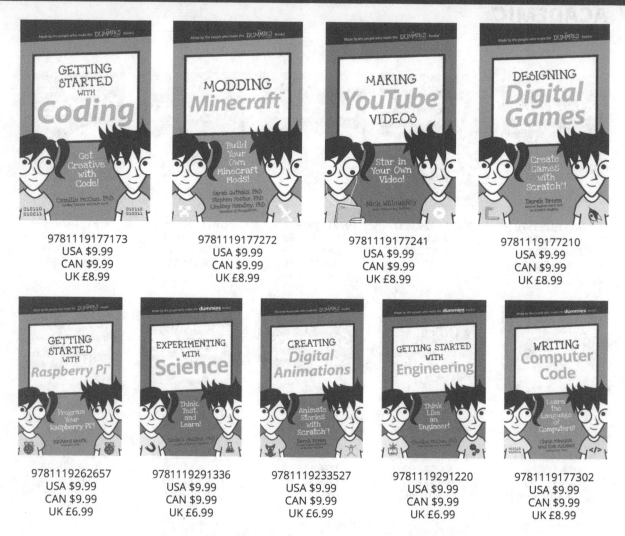

GETTING STARTED WITH Coding
Get Creative with Code!
Camille McCue, PhD
9781119177173
USA $9.99
CAN $9.99
UK £8.99

MODDING Minecraft™
Build Your Own Minecraft Mods!
Sarah Guthals, PhD
Stephen Foster, PhD
Lindsey Handley, PhD
9781119177272
USA $9.99
CAN $9.99
UK £8.99

MAKING YouTube VIDEOS
Star in Your Own Video!
Nick Willoughby
9781119177241
USA $9.99
CAN $9.99
UK £8.99

DESIGNING Digital Games
Create Games with Scratch™!
Derek Breen
9781119177210
USA $9.99
CAN $9.99
UK £8.99

GETTING STARTED WITH Raspberry Pi™
Program Your Raspberry Pi!
Richard Wentk
9781119262657
USA $9.99
CAN $9.99
UK £6.99

EXPERIMENTING WITH Science
Think, Test, and Learn!
9781119291336
USA $9.99
CAN $9.99
UK £6.99

CREATING Digital Animations
Animate Stories with Scratch™!
Derek Breen
9781119233527
USA $9.99
CAN $9.99
UK £6.99

GETTING STARTED WITH Engineering
Think Like an Engineer!
9781119291220
USA $9.99
CAN $9.99
UK £6.99

WRITING Computer Code
Learn the Language of Computers!
Chris Minnick and Eva Holland
9781119177302
USA $9.99
CAN $9.99
UK £8.99

Unleash Their Creativity

dummies.com

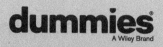

dummies®
A Wiley Brand